Emotional and Behavioral Problems of Young Children

The Guilford Practical Intervention in the Schools Series

Kenneth W. Merrell, Series Editor

Helping Students Overcome Depression and Anxiety: A Practical Guide
Kenneth W. Merrell

Emotional and Behavioral Problems of Young Children:
Effective Interventions in the Preschool and Kindergarten Years
Gretchen A. Gimpel and Melissa L. Holland

Conducting School-Based Functional Behavioral Assessments:
A Practitioner's Guide
T. Steuart Watson and Mark W. Steege

Emotional and Behavioral Problems of Young Children

Effective Interventions in the Preschool and Kindergarten Years

GRETCHEN A. GIMPEL
MELISSA L. HOLLAND

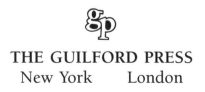

THE GUILFORD PRESS
New York   London

© 2003 The Guilford Press
A Division of Guilford Publications, Inc.
72 Spring St., New York, NY 10012
www.guilford.com

Printed in Canada

This book is printed on acid-free paper.

Last digit is print number: 9 8 7 6 5 4 3 2 1

Library of Congress Cataloging-in-Publication Data

Gimpel, Gretchen A.
   Emotional and behavioral problems of young children : effective interventions in the preschool and kindergarten years / Gretchen A. Gimpel, Melissa L. Holland.
      p. cm. — (The Guilford practical intervention in the schools series)
Includes bibliographical references and index.
   ISBN 1-57230-861-3 (pbk.)
1. Adjustment disorders in children.   2. Preschool children—Mental health.   3. Kindergarten.
I. Holland, Melissa L.   II. Title.   III. Series.
RJ506.A33 G565 2003
618.92′89—dc21

                                                 2002152748

About the Authors

Gretchen A. Gimpel, PhD, is an Associate Professor of Psychology at Utah State University, where she is the Program Coordinator of the NASP-approved MS program in School Psychology and is on the program faculty of the Combined (School/Clinical/Counseling) APA-accredited PhD program. Dr. Gimpel is a licensed psychologist and certified school psychologist. She teaches core child therapy and assessment courses for psychology graduate students. Dr. Gimpel also coordinates child therapy services within the Psychology Department's Community Clinic and conducts an ongoing treatment study for children with ADHD and their families. Her publications and professional presentations are in the area of child behavior problems and family issues as related to child behaviors.

Melissa L. Holland, PhD, is currently in private practice in Sacramento, California, specializing in work with children, adolescents, and their families. She is both a licensed clinical psychologist and a certified school psychologist. Dr. Holland previously worked in mental health clinics; community, child, and family agencies; a major medical center; and a Head Start program providing assessment and intervention services to children and their families. Her publications are in the area of child and family mental health. Dr. Holland recently developed and published a rating scale (with Gretchen A. Gimpel and Kenneth W. Merrell as coauthors) to assess for ADHD in the childhood population (the ADHD Symptoms Rating Scale; ADHD-SRS).

Preface

This book is intended to provide child-focused mental health providers with information on how to address common emotional and behavioral problems exhibited by preschool- and kindergarten-age children (ages 3–6). Our main focus is to provide practical and effective interventions that can easily be implemented by clinicians working in educational settings, as well as by clinical psychologists and other mental health providers working with children in nonschool settings. In addition, we emphasize working with parents of young children who are exhibiting behaviors of concern. Although some techniques for working individually with children are covered, it is our belief that parents are instrumental in resolving problems young children are experiencing, given the fact that preschool children spend much of their days with their parents.

Although preschool and kindergarten children may not be diagnosed with specific disorders or classified according to specific special education categories, they may still exhibit a number of behavioral and emotional problems that cause concern for their parents and teachers. In addition, research has consistently shown that approximately 50% of children who exhibit problems in the preschool years continue to have problems into elementary school, and even later. Thus it is important to provide early intervention to decrease the potential negative long-term effects of these difficulties. This book provides clinicians with interventions that have been shown to be effective, or show promise of being effective, with young children. All interventions discussed are based on treatment-outcome research, to the extent possible. However, for some of the areas covered in this book, there is little research to guide effective practice specifically with preschool- and kindergarten-age children. Thus not all interventions covered in this book should be considered empirically supported; however, the interventions discussed are considered best practice, based on current information and research.

The book begins with an overview of childhood emotional and behavioral problems and how these are likely to manifest during the preschool and kindergarten years. Also discussed in Chapter 1 are correlates of these problems and information related to the continuity of such difficulties. Following this introductory chapter, information on assessment methods is provided: Both norm-referenced assessment measures (rating scales) as well as other types of assessment methods (interviews, observations) are discussed. This chapter specifically focuses on the use of these measures and techniques with the young child in mind. The remaining four chapters cover interventions for specific areas of concern. Chapter 3 covers the treatment of externalizing problems in young children (e.g., ADHD, conduct problems); in this chapter, parent training is discussed extensively. Chapter 4 covers interventions for internalizing problems (i.e., anxiety and depression); the specific anxiety disorders most likely to be diagnosed in the preschool years are highlighted (e.g., specific phobias, separation anxiety disorder). Chapter 5 reviews the treatment of "everyday problems," such as those involving toileting issues (i.e., enuresis and encopresis), sleeping problems (e.g., frequent night wakings), and feeding problems (e.g., children who are "picky" eaters). Because of the nature of these problems, the interventions discussed in this chapter are primarily focused on working with parents. In Chapter 6, interventions for children who have been abused are discussed. Posttraumatic stress disorder is highlighted in this chapter, as this disorder is a frequent consequence of abuse.

Each chapter contains parent handouts, assessment tools, and other reproducible materials. Many of these materials are similar to those that appear in other sources, but we have found the versions presented here to be particularly helpful in our work with young children.

This book will be a helpful, practical resource for individuals working with preschool- and kindergarten-age children exhibiting emotional and behavioral problems. Although some of the interventions may seem fairly straightforward, they should be implemented by individuals with training and expertise in child development and basic knowledge of therapeutic interventions. Individuals who would likely find this book useful include school psychologists working in the preschool and kindergarten setting; psychologists and master's-level mental health professionals in private practice who provide services to young children; pediatricians with a strong background in behavioral interventions; and other professionals with child-focused training. In addition, this book would be a useful resource in graduate child therapy didactic and practicum courses.

Contents

1. **Introduction to Behavioral, Social, and Emotional Problems of Young Children** 1

Overview of Disorders 2
  Externalizing Problems 2
  Internalizing Problems 4
  Other Problems 6
  Abuse and Neglect 7
  Pervasive Developmental Disorders 8
  Summary of Problems 10
Prevalence and Definition Issues 10
Stability of Behavior Problems 13
Predictors of Problems 14
  Predictors of Externalizing Problems 14
  Predictors of Internalizing Problems 17
Chapter Summary/Purpose of Book 18

2. **Assessment of Mental Health Issues in Preschool and Kindergarten Children** 19

Interviews with Parents and Teachers 20
  Parent/Caregiver Interviews 20
  Teacher/Daycare Worker Interviews 28
Interviews with Young Children 29
  Rapport Building/Initial Information Gathering 30
  Context of the Interview 32
  Mental Status Examination 34
Rating Scales 35
  Child Behavior Checklist and Teacher's Report Form 35
  Behavior Assessment System for Children 36
  Conners' Rating Scales 37
  Preschool and Kindergarten Behavior Scales 38
  Eyberg Child Behavior Inventory 38

Social Skills Rating System   39
Attention Deficit Disorder Evaluation Scale   39
ADHD-Symptoms Rating Scale   40
ADHD Rating Scale–IV   40
Limitations of Rating Scales   41
Direct Observation   41
Defining Observable Behaviors   42
Structured Observations   42
Formal Observations   49
Chapter Summary   49

3. **Treatment of Externalizing/Acting-Out Problems**   50

Parent Training as an Intervention for Externalizing Problems   51
Overview   51
Initial Considerations   52
Conducting Parent Training   53
Group Parent Training   74
Preschool- and Kindergarten-Based Behavioral Intervention Programs   75
Social Skills Interventions   80
Prevention/Early Intervention Programs   82
Chapter Summary   85

4. **Treatment of Internalizing Problems**   86

Overview of Common Fears, Phobias, and Anxieties   86
Specific Phobia   88
Separation Anxiety   88
Posttraumatic Stress Disorder   89
Treatment of Anxiety Problems in Young Children   89
Specific Phobia   90
Separation Anxiety, Including Early School or Daycare Refusal   100
Selective Mutism   105
Overview of Depressive Symptoms   107
Prevention of Childhood Depression   108
Treatment of Depressive Symptoms   108
Chapter Summary   113

5. **Managing and Preventing Everyday Problems**   114

Toileting   114
Toilet Training   114
Enuresis   116
Encopresis   125
Feeding/Eating Problems and Interventions   130
Treatment of Typical Feeding Problems   130
Pica   134
Rumination   134
Sleep Problems   135
Problems Initiating Sleep   136
Arousal Disorders   143
Chapter Summary   146

6. Working with Young Children Who Have Been Abused 147

Overview of Physical, Sexual, and Emotional Abuse and Neglect   147
Effects of Child Abuse   149
  Physical Effects   149
  Psychological Effects   149
Interventions for Young Children Who Have Been Abused   152
Posttraumatic Stress Disorder   156
  Treatment of PTSD in Young Children   156
Prevention Methods for Parents and Teachers   158
Chapter Summary   160

References   161

Index   173

Emotional and Behavioral Problems of Young Children

1

Introduction to Behavioral, Social, and Emotional Problems of Young Children

Over the past several decades there has been increased interest in the social and emotional development of preschool- and kindergarten-age children. Prior to this shift in focus, the common belief among parents, professionals, and researchers was that difficulties exhibited by young children were due to their developmental immaturity and that they would outgrow their problems. It is certainly true that the preschool and kindergarten years are a time of tremendous development and change, so some instability in behaviors is to be expected. However, it has become increasingly clear that many children who exhibit emotional and behavior problems in their early childhood years will continue to have such problems over time and perhaps throughout their adolescent and even adult years.

With the increasing recognition that emotional and behavioral problems often do *not* decline naturally, there has been an increased focus on intervention and prevention efforts geared toward preschool and kindergarten children. This book provides an overview of interventions that have been found to be effective or appear promising for use with young children. This first chapter briefly reviews emotional and behavior problems that may be exhibited by children during the preschool and kindergarten years as well as the prevalence of these disorders. An overview of the research on the continuity of such problems and the predictors of these problems concludes this chapter. Chapter 2 presents information regarding the assessment of young children suspected of having emotional or behavior problems. Each of the remaining four chapters presents detailed information regarding interventions for specific problems that are commonly seen in the preschool and kindergarten years. Chapter 3 covers externalizing/acting-out behaviors associated with conduct problems, oppositional behavior, and attention-deficit/hyperactivity disorder (ADHD). Chapter 4 covers internalizing problems such as fears, anxieties, and depression. Chapter 5 reviews treatments for everyday problems that are commonly seen in preschool- and kindergarten-age children, including toileting problems, feeding issues, and sleep difficulties. In Chapter 6, interventions for children who have been abused are described.

OVERVIEW OF DISORDERS

Emotional and behavioral problems of children are typically divided into two general categories: externalizing and internalizing problems. *Externalizing problems* are outer-directed and involve acting-out, defiant, and noncompliant behaviors. *Internalizing problems* are more inner-directed and involve withdrawal, depression, and anxiety. In addition, young children commonly exhibit problems that do not fall within either of these general domains (e.g., difficulties with sleep schedules, eating problems, and toilet-training–related problems). In the sections that follow, brief descriptions of the more common emotional and behavioral problems of the early childhood years are provided. These problems are summarized in Table 1.1.

Externalizing Problems

There are three generally recognized externalizing disorders: attention-deficit/hyperactivity disorder (ADHD), oppositional defiant disorder (ODD), and conduct disorder (CD). Although each of these disorders can be diagnosed in young children, it is rare for a young child to receive the diagnosis of CD, given its more serious nature. However, as will be discussed later, ODD (often considered a milder form of CD) is one of the more common disorders diagnosed during the preschool and kindergarten years. Diagnoses of ADHD are becoming more common during the preschool and kindergarten years, although there is still much debate about whether this disorder should be diagnosed in young children, and if diagnosed, how that determination should be made.

TABLE 1.1. Common Emotional and Behavioral Problems

Externalizing problems	Other problems
Attention-deficit/hyperactivity disorder	Selective mutism
Predominately inattentive type	Enuresis
Predominately hyperactive–impulsive type	Encopresis
Combined type	Feeding disorder of infancy or early childhood
Oppositional defiant disorder	Pica
Conduct disorder	Rumination
	Sleep problems
Internalizing problems	
	Disorders linked to abuse and neglect
Separation anxiety disorder	
Generalized anxiety disorder	Posttraumatic stress disorder
Social phobia	Reactive attachment disorder
Obsessive–compulsive disorder	
Specific phobia	Pervasive developmental disorders
Panic disorder	
Major depressive disorder	Autism
Dysthymic disorder	Asperger's disorder
	Rett's disorder
	Childhood disintegrative disorder

Over the past several years, ADHD has received increasing attention in both the research and popular literature. Much of this attention has focused on school-age children, but increasingly researchers are studying ADHD as a syndrome that may be diagnosable in the preschool and kindergarten years. ADHD, which has a prevalence rate of 3–5% in the general school-age population and is more common in boys than girls (American Psychiatric Association, 1994), is defined as "a persistent pattern of inattention and/or hyperactivity–impulsivity that is more frequent and severe than is typically observed in individuals at a comparable level of development" (American Psychiatric Association, 1994, p. 78). The fourth edition of the Diagnostic and Statistical Manual of Mental Disorders (DSM-IV; American Psychiatric Association, 1994) specifies that symptoms must be present prior to age 7; thus symptoms must first be observed by the late preschool/early elementary school years. Additional diagnostic criteria for ADHD include the presence of symptoms across at least two settings, and evidence that symptoms interfere with functioning. Obviously, preschool and kindergarten children are, by nature, less attentive and more active than are older children. The DSM-IV acknowledges that "hyperactivity may vary with the individual's age and developmental level, and the diagnosis should be made cautiously in young children" (American Psychiatric Association, 1994, p. 79), and that "it is especially difficult to establish this diagnosis in children younger than 4 or 5 years" (p. 81).

There are currently three subtypes of ADHD defined in the DSM-IV: ADHD, predominately inattentive type (in which the child shows at least six of nine inattentive symptoms but less than six hyperactive–impulsive symptoms); ADHD, predominately hyperactive–impulsive type (in which the child shows at least six of nine hyperactive–impulsive symptoms but less than six inattentive symptoms); and ADHD, combined type (in which the child shows at least six symptoms of both inattention and hyperactivity–impulsivity). Researchers have consistently found support for the two-factor configuration of ADHD (inattention and hyperactivity–impulsivity) in school-age children, and the presence of the three subtypes (i.e., hyperactive–impulsive, inattentive, and combined) has been validated in a sample of children ages 4–6 (Lahey et al., 1998). However, it is still unclear whether this two-factor model is the most appropriate one for preschool-age children or whether ADHD is better conceptualized as a unidimensional construct in young children. It is generally agreed that there is a developmental progression of symptoms in either case. Preschool and kindergarten children tend to exhibit more hyperactive and impulsive behaviors than inattentive behaviors. In fact, the majority of diagnoses for the predominately hyperactive–impulsive type of ADHD are in children age 6 or younger. Inattentive behaviors, either alone or in combination with previously exhibited hyperactive–impulsive behaviors, begin to appear around the time children enter school. Thus, children over age 6 are most likely to receive a combined-type diagnosis or a predominately inattentive-type diagnosis. By adolescence many children with ADHD no longer have the overt hyperactive symptoms and display mostly inattentive symptoms (American Psychiatric Association, 1994; Lahey et al., 1998).

ODD is defined in the DSM-IV as "a recurrent pattern of negativistic, defiant, disobedient, and hostile behavior toward authority figures" (American Psychiatric Association, 1994, p. 91). ODD has a general prevalence rate of 2–16% and, like ADHD, is more common in males than females, at least until adolescence. Symptoms of ODD generally appear by the time the child is in early elementary school and typically first appear in the home setting (American Psychiatric Association, 1994).

A substantial number of children with ODD eventually develop the more serious behavior disorder of CD. In fact, many researchers believe that ODD is a developmental precursor to CD, and the two disorders are often discussed together as "conduct problems." Children who exhibit conduct problems at an early age often progress from oppositional behaviors to low-level CD behaviors (e.g., lying, bullying), and then to more severe CD behaviors, such as vandalism and fire setting (Loeber, Green, Lahey, Frick, & McBurnett, 2000).

CD is defined as "a repetitive and persistent pattern of behavior in which the basic rights of others or major age-appropriate societal norms or rules are violated" (American Psychiatric Association, 1994, p. 85). Two subtypes of CD are delineated in the DSM-IV: a childhood-onset type, in which at least one symptom of CD is present prior to age 10; and an adolescent-onset type, in which no symptoms are present prior to age 10. The onset of CD typically does not occur in the preschool or kindergarten years. The DSM indicates that CD may have an onset "as early as age 5–6 years but is usually in late childhood or early adolescence" (American Psychiatric Association, 1994, p. 89). Although it is unlikely that young children will be diagnosed with CD, it is worthwhile for clinicians working with preschool- and kindergarten-age children to have a good understanding of both ODD and CD, given the link between the two.

Internalizing Problems

Internalizing problems tend to be less commonly diagnosed than externalizing problems in the early childhood years although, as is discussed below, several research groups have found that internalizing and externalizing symptoms are equally common in young children when rating scales such as the Child Behavior Checklist are used to identify symptoms. Although it may be rare for a preschool- or kindergarten-age child to exhibit internalizing symptoms to the extent to which a formal diagnosis is warranted, high levels of internalizing symptoms may still indicate a need for clinical intervention.

Although the DSM-IV lists the three externalizing disorders under the category of "Disorders Usually First Diagnosed in Infancy, Childhood, or Adolescence," only one internalizing disorder is addressed in this chapter. Certainly children may be diagnosed with disorders not listed in this section, but we believe it can be problematic to apply criteria developed primarily for adults to a young population.

Separation anxiety disorder (SAD) is the only internalizing disorder listed in the childhood chapter in the DSM-IV. Although other anxiety disorders were listed in this chapter in the previous edition of the DSM (i.e., overanxious disorder and avoidant disorder), these disorders were subsumed under other categories in the general anxiety disorders chapter. SAD involves "excessive anxiety concerning separation from the home or from those to whom the person is attached" (American Psychiatric Association, 1994, p. 110). Children with SAD exhibit a great deal of distress when separated from their caregivers, or even when separation is imminent but has yet to occur. These children typically fear that some harm will come to their caregivers or that something bad will happen to them (e.g., kidnapping). They attempt to avoid separation and may exhibit "clingy" behavior with their caregivers (Albano, Chorpita, & Barlow, 2003; American Psychiatric Association, 1994). As with all disorders, this concern must be atypical for the child's developmental level and cause the child significant distress or impairment in functioning. SAD may have an onset in the preschool or kindergarten years; if the onset is prior to age 6 it is considered to be "early onset" (American Psychiatric Association, 1994). Some separation anxiety is part of typical development for children up to about age 6, so for a young child to receive a diagnosis of SAD, the anxiety must be more severe than the anxiety experienced by other children his/her age.

In addition to SAD, children may be diagnosed with any of the other anxiety disorders defined in the DSM-IV (e.g., specific phobia, social phobia, generalized anxiety disorder, obsessive–compulsive disorder). These disorders are briefly discussed below. Many young children with anxieties, though, will not meet criteria for a specific disorder. Instead, they may exhibit general symptoms of anxiety, including fearfulness, shyness, and so on. If these symptoms are severe enough (whether or not a formal anxiety disorder is diagnosed or not), treatment should be considered.

Generalized anxiety disorder (GAD; formerly known as overanxious disorder [OAD] in children) involves "excessive anxiety and worry . . . about a number of events or activities" (American Psychiatric Association, 1994, p. 432). The prevalence rate of OAD in children was estimated at 3%, with higher rates reported in adolescents. Although cases of OAD were reported in preschool- and kindergarten-age children, the typical onset was not until later childhood (Albano et al., 2003). Given that the application of GAD to children is relatively new, information on this disorder specifically in children (particularly in preschool- and kindergarten-age children) is still lacking.

Social phobia involves a "marked and persistent fear of social or performance situations in which embarrassment may occur" (American Psychiatric Association, 1994, p. 411). Children with social phobia typically have few friends and often attempt to avoid social interactions. Young children may exhibit social inhibition (being timid/withdrawn in new situations); however, social phobia is rarely diagnosed until later childhood or adolescence (Albano et al., 2003).

Obsessive–compulsive disorder (OCD) involves repeated obsessions or compulsions that are time consuming and cause distress (American Psychiatric Association, 1994). Children's obsessions may include contamination fears or dire religious or aggressive themes; their compulsions often involve washing, checking, and arranging. Although there have been reports of OCD in preschool- and kindergarten-age children, the onset more typically occurs in the later childhood years. However, boys do seem to have an earlier onset than girls (Albano et al., 2003).

Specific phobias involve "marked and persistent fear of clearly discernible, circumscribed objects or situations" (American Psychiatric Association, 1994, p. 405). Upon exposure to the object or situation, the person experiences an anxiety response; often the feared object is avoided to prevent the anxiety response. Adults must recognize that their fear is excessive for the diagnosis to apply; however, children do not need to have this realization in order to receive a diagnosis of specific phobia. Although fears are common in young children, specific, diagnosable phobias are less common, with prevalence estimates typically being under 10%. Children's fears tend to change over time; fears in the preschool years often involve separation from parents, noises, the dark, and animals. These fears are considered developmentally normal, unless the response is much more severe than would be expected in a given situation. As children age, they tend to develop fears more related to academic and social events (Morris & Kratochwill, 1998).

Panic disorder is defined as the occurrence of repeated panic attacks (a short but intense period of fear or discomfort). Until recently it was believed that panic disorder did not occur in children, but researchers have begun to identify cases of this disorder in school-age children. Given the cognitive components of this disorder (concern about having a panic attack, worry about what the attacks mean), it is more difficult to identify this disorder in children (Albano et al., 2003), and it is unlikely that this disorder would be diagnosed in young children.

Although there is no specific childhood version of depression, children may be diagnosed with the depressive disorders outlined in the DSM-IV, including major depressive disorder and dysthymic disorder. Although there are no specific depressive criteria for children, the DSM-IV does note that instead of having a "depressed mood," children may exhibit an "irritable mood." Symptoms of depression change with age, and younger children are more likely than older children to exhibit somatic complaints, irritability, and social withdrawal (American Psychiatric Association, 1994, p. 327). Rates of depression in children have been estimated to be between 0.4% and 2.5% for major depression, and between 0.6% and 1.7% for dysthymic disorder. Although in adolescence and adulthood the rate of depression is significantly higher in females than males, prior to this time, rates are approximately equal (Birmaher et al., 1996). The prevalence rate of depression in preschool- and kindergarten-age children is unclear, given the limited number of studies that have included children in this age range, but the prevalence is likely below 1% (Hammen & Rudolph, 2003).

Other Problems

In addition to the externalizing and internalizing disorders, there are a number of other problems with which children can present for treatment. Some of the more common "other problems" seen in preschool children including selective mutism, toileting difficulties, feeding problems, and sleeping problems are reviewed here.

Selective mutism involves a "persistent failure to speak in specific social situations (e.g., school, with playmates) where speaking is expected, despite speaking in other situations" (American Psychiatric Association, 1994, p. 114). This disorder is sometimes categorized as an internalizing disorder due to the fact that it is often considered to have anxiety as a precipitator. (Treatment of this disorder is discussed with the other anxiety disorders in Chapter 4.) The onset of selective mutism typically occurs during the preschool years; it is fairly rare and often does not continue longer than a couple months (American Psychiatric Association, 1994). However, for children in preschool or kindergarten, in particular, this disorder can be quite impairing and should be treated.

Toileting problems (enuresis and encopresis) are also commonly seen in young children. Enuresis is characterized by the voiding of urine in either one's clothes during the daytime (diurnal enuresis) or in one's bed during the night (nocturnal enuresis). According to the DSM-IV, children must be at least 5 years old to be diagnosed with enuresis. Nocturnal enuresis, in particular, is quite common through the early elementary school years, and thus treatment is not typically warranted until after the preschool years. Encopresis, the passage of feces in inappropriate places, is less common than enuresis. A child must be at least 4 to receive a diagnosis of encopresis, and the inappropriate soiling must occur on a regular basis (American Psychiatric Association, 1994).

Feeding disorders covered in the DSM-IV include pica (eating nonfood items), rumination (regurgitation and rechewing of food), and feeding disorder of infancy or early childhood (failure to eat adequately to gain weight). However, young children often exhibit problems related to feeding and eating that do not meet criteria for a formal disorder. Children may be "picky eaters" or have other issues related to eating (e.g., behavior problems while eating, such as spitting out food) that are not diagnosable disorders. Although not meeting the criteria for a clinical disorder, these issues can still be highly problematic for parents, and treatment is often warranted.

Sleep problems are also commonly reported by parents of young children. It is estimated that at least 25% of preschool-age children have sleep problems, and many of these children continue to have problems for a number of years. In fact, having sleep problems as a child may predict the presence of sleep problems in adulthood. Common sleep problems in young children include nighttime wakings and problems initiating sleep. Children with disorders such as autism and other developmental disabilities exhibit sleep problems even more frequently (Durand, Mindell, Mapstone, & Gernet-Dott, 1998).

Abuse and Neglect

Although abuse and neglect are not problems children *exhibit*, they are, unfortunately, problems that young children experience. The outcomes of abuse and neglect are quite variable and dependent upon a number of factors. Clearly, though, many children suffer a number of adverse outcomes due to abuse and neglect. Some of the more common DSM-IV disorders that may result from abuse and neglect are posttraumatic stress disorder and reactive attachment disorder. Children who have been abused are also at greater risk than their nonabused counterparts for almost any psychological problem.

Posttraumatic stress disorder (PTSD) and the shorter-duration acute stress disorder (ASD) are classified as anxiety disorders in the DSM-IV, although there is controversy regarding whether these disorders belong in this section. PTSD occurs following exposure to a traumatic event that involved "actual or threatened death or serious injury, or other threat to one's physical integrity" (American Psychiatric Association, 1994, p. 424). The reaction to this event must have involved "fear, helplessness or horror;" in children this response can be expressed through "disorganized or agitated behavior" (American Psychiatric Association, 1994 p. 424). In the not-too-distant past, it was assumed that stressful life events did not affect children in any significant, long-lasting manner. That view has changed and during the past decade, there has been a large increase in the number of studies focused on PTSD in children. Current research supports the application of PTSD criteria to children, including preschool- and kindergarten-age children. Some of the more common symptoms of PTSD in young children include bad dreams, experiencing distress in response to reminders of the event, reenacting the trauma via play, and trauma-specific fears. It has been estimated that 39% of preschool-age children exposed to trauma meet the criteria for PTSD (Fletcher, 2003).

Reactive attachment disorder, by definition, begins prior to age 5 and involves some impairment in the ability to form attachments and relate socially to others. Children may be diagnosed with one of two subtypes of the disorder. The inhibited type involves a lack of initiation or response to social situations; the disinhibited type involves indiscriminate sociablity. Reactive attachment disorder occurs following neglectful or pathogenic (e.g., abusive) care of the child (American Psychiatric Association, 1994).

Pervasive Developmental Disorders

Other disorders that often are first diagnosed in the preschool years are the pervasive developmental disorders, including autism, Asperger's disorder, childhood disintegrative disorder, and Rett's disorder. These disorders involve delays and impairments across a number of developmental areas, such as social interactions, communication, and behavior. Given the complex nature of these disorders and their treatment, we have chosen not to address them in depth in this book; it is our belief that we would be unable to adequately cover these disorders in a relatively short, practically oriented treatment manual. These disorders are discussed briefly below; for those desiring more comprehensive coverage of treatment issues, we recommend obtaining other resources.

Autism is the best known and most researched of the pervasive developmental disorders. According to the DSM-IV definition of autism, children must have impairments in social interactions and communication and exhibit restricted/stereotyped behaviors and interests (American Psychiatric Association, 1994). The impairments in social interactions involve a wide range of behaviors, including difficulties engaging in (1) age-appropriate play (particularly, symbolic play), (2) social imitation and responsive behaviors in relation to emotions and social cues of others, and (3) nonverbal social behaviors (Klinger, Dawson, & Renner, 2003). Attachment traditionally has been seen as a problem for children with autism; however, research suggests that many children with autism do form secure attachments with their caregivers (Capps, Sigman, & Mundy, 1994). The impairments in communication involve significant difficulties with speech and the use of language. Approximately 50% of children with autism never develop speech. Of those children who do develop some speech abilities, their speech is typically odd and characterized by echolalia, unusual prosody, and pronoun reversal. In particular, children with autism have difficulties with speech in social situations, where they may include unnecessary details, change topics frequently, and tend to be too concrete and literal in their interpretations of what others say. The atypical behaviors seen in children with autism involve stereotyped routines, preoccupation with objects, repetitive movements, and self-stimulatory behaviors. In addition to these primary symptoms of autism, the majority of children with this disorder have low cognitive abilities (Klinger et al., 2003).

To be diagnosed with autism, children must first show symptoms of the disorder prior to age 3 (American Psychiatric Association, 1994). Autism is more common in males than females and has an estimated prevalence rate of 4–5 in every 10,000 children. Recent literature, though, has suggested that the prevalence of autism may actually be higher than this figure. A recent report suggests that the rate may be as high as 7.5 per 10,000. According to this report, this revised rate reflects better identification of autism and not an actual increase in the number of children with autism (National Research Council, 2001). The exact cause of autism is unknown, and it is likely that there are different causes for different children. Research has focused on biological factors, including complications during pregnancy or birth, neurotransmitter imbalances, and brain structure abnormalities. Autism does have a genetic component, with high concordance rates for identical twins (Klinger & Dawson, 1996).

Although there have been a number of proposed interventions for autism, many of these have little or no empirical support. Early and intensive educational services aimed at helping children acquire basic skills are the only interventions with significant empirical support and seem to be extremely important in improving the functioning of children with autism (American Academy of Child and Adolescent Psychiatry, 1999).

Asperger's disorder is another of the pervasive developmental disorders that has received increased attention over the past decade. Asperger's involves impairments in social interactions and the exhibition of restricted/stereotyped behaviors as does autism. However, unlike children with autism, children with Asperger's do not show a significant delay in language skills. In addition, children with Asperger's do not experience impairments in cognitive development and adaptive skills, as do many children with autism (American Psychiatric Association, 1994). The diagnosis of Asperger's has caused considerable controversy, as there are some researchers in the field of pervasive developmental disorders who see Asperger's as one end of the continuum of autism and not as a separate disorder (Klinger & Dawson, 1996). It is unlikely that this controversy will be resolved any time soon.

Childhood disintegrative disorder (CDD) and Rett's disorder have received considerably less attention in the research literature. CDD is characterized by a regression in functioning following at least 2 years of normal functioning. This regression must be seen in at least two of the following areas: expressive–receptive language, social skills–adaptive behavior, bladder–bowel control, play, and motor skills. In addition, abnormalities must be noted in at least two of the areas associated with autism (social interactions, communication, restricted behaviors) (American Psychiatric Association, 1994). CDD appears to be quite rare and is less prevalent than autism. Although many children with CDD experience seizures, no specific neurological abnormality has yet been associated with the disorder (Tanguay, 2000).

Rett's disorder also involves deterioration in functioning following a period of normal development. Children with this disorder develop normally for at least the first 5 months of life and then experience a deceleration in head growth, loss of purposeful hand movements, loss of social engagement, poorly coordinated gait, and impaired expressive and receptive language (American Psychiatric Association, 1994). Rett's disorder is relatively rare and gender-linked, with an estimated prevalence rate of 1 in 10,000–15,000 females (Tanguay, 2000). Although there have been some reports of males with symptoms similar to those seen in females with Rett's, for the most part this disorder appears to be specific to females. Rett's is likely caused by a gene on the X chromosome (mutations in the MeCP2 gene have been noted), and pregnancies involving males with such a defect would most likely result in a miscarriage (Tanguay, 2000).

Summary of Problems

As should be clear from the disorders reviewed above, there are a number of social/ emotional/behavioral problems that young children may exhibit. Although our review of disorders was organized around DSM categories, it should be noted that many preschool and kindergarten children who are referred for emotional and behavioral problems will not receive a diagnosis of a specific disorder. In many instances, a full diagnostic assessment may not be needed or warranted. For example, a clinician may choose not to attach a diagnosis to a preschool or kindergarten child who is exhibiting general acting-out behavior problems. Instead the clinician may complete an assessment (e.g., parent interview, rating scale) to gather information on the nature of the problems but not tie the assessment results to a formal diagnosis if it is not required for treatment purposes (e.g., insurance reimbursement, access to services). In other situations, a full diagnostic assessment may be undertaken, and the child may not meet the criteria for a formal diagnosis, though the child may still exhibit sufficient problems of concern to the parent or teacher to warrant intervention. It is important that clinicians not fall into the trap of thinking that a diagnosis is necessary in order for treatment to be provided. Although a formal diagnosis may help guide treatment selection, it is more important that the specific behaviors of concern be identified for treatment selection than it is that a DSM-IV diagnosis be assigned. However, for insurance reimbursement, actual diagnoses typically are necessary. In these cases, when the child does not meet criteria for any specific disorder but is exhibiting symptoms that significantly interfere with functioning, and therefore warrant intervention, he/she may be diagnosed with the disorder of infancy, childhood or adolescence not otherwise specified.

PREVALENCE AND DEFINITION ISSUES

Although the previous section cited prevalence estimates of disorders in children, the prevalence of emotional and behavioral problems in preschool- and kindergarten-age children is largely unknown, due to a lack of research in this area as well as difficulties defining psychological disorders in young children. In fact, the epidemiology of disorders in this population has received little attention until relatively recently. Parents frequently report concerns regarding their children's behaviors, with half to two-thirds of parents of infants and toddlers expressing some concern. Common concerns of parents focus on child management difficulties (the child is "difficult," "demanding," or "overactive"), eating problems, and sleep problems (Mathiesen & Sanson, 2000; Stallard, 1993). Of course, not all of these parental concerns translate into diagnosable disorders or are even severe enough to cause parents to seek treatment for their children.

Studies investigating the prevalence of disorders in preschool- and kindergarten-age children typically use rating scales such as the Child Behavior Checklist (reviewed in Chapter 2), the categorical criteria in the *Diagnostic and Statistical Manual of Mental Disorders,* currently in its fourth edition (DSM-IV; American Psychiatric Association, 1994), or a combination of these two methods. When using rating scales, children are typically classified as having a significant problem if they score above a certain cutoff score (e.g., above the 90th percentile).

The DSM system utilizes a multiaxial approach to diagnosis. The majority of clinical diagnoses and all of the disorders discussed in this text fall on Axis I. Axis II includes mental retardation and the personality disorders. Medical conditions, psychosocial stressors, and overall functioning are coded on the remaining three axes. When determining if a child meets criteria for a DSM diagnosis, the criteria are compared to the child's symptoms. For behavior to be considered as symptomatic, it must be atypical for the child's level of development. In addition, symptoms must be causing the child some impairment (e.g., problems with social relationships, conflict with parents). There is considerable debate as to whether DSM criteria and diagnoses should be applied to young children. Arguments against the use of DSM with young children include: (1) The symptoms are too subjective, (2) the symptoms do not apply to preschool- and kindergarten-age children, and (3) the reliability and validity of the diagnoses have not been established with young children. Although research on the use of the DSM system in young children is limited, there is some evidence to support the validity of certain DSM diagnoses (i.e., oppositional defiant disorder and conduct disorder) in preschool-age children (Keenan & Wakschlag, 2002). It is likely that as researchers increasingly focus their attention on this age range, additional studies examining the validity of the DSM system for use with preschool-age children will be conducted. However, even with additional research, the controversy over the use of the DSM will no doubt continue. Nevertheless, the DSM remains one of the most common diagnostic tools applied to children of all ages.

In one of the first studies to apply DSM criteria to young children, 21 of 100 3-year-old children met criteria for a DSM-III disorder, with the most common disorders being separation anxiety disorder and oppositional defiant disorder (Earls, 1982). In an early study of 100 clinic-referred preschool children, 60% were reported to have a DSM-III diagnosis. Adjustment disorders were the most common problems, followed by ADHD and conduct problems (Kashani, Horwitz, Ray, & Reid, 1986).

Several more recent studies examining the prevalence of behavior problems in young children have used both DSM criteria and Child Behavior Checklist score cutoffs. In one such study, 8.3% of 2- to 5-year-old children were considered to have a behavior problem when using a cutoff score of 90% on the CBCL. The overall rate of DSM-III-R disorders in this same sample was 21.4% (9.1% of which were considered severe). Across these two methods of defining disorders, boys were more likely to exhibit problem behaviors than were girls. Although internalizing and externalizing problems were equally common on CBCL ratings, the disruptive behavior disorders were the most common DSM-defined problems. Oppositional defiant disorder was the most common diagnosis (16.8% total; 8.1% severe), and ADHD was diagnosed in 2% of the sample (usually as a co-occurring disorder). Internalizing disorders were less prevalent, with rates below 1% for the individual anxiety disorders and depression; however, when anxiety disorders were combined, the overall prevalence rate was around 2% (Lavigne et al., 1996).

A study of low-income 4- and 5-year-old children found somewhat higher rates of DSM-III-R disorders, with 14.9% exhibiting an externalizing disorder and 14.9% exhibiting an internalizing disorder. Oppositional defiant disorder was again the most common diagnosis (12.6%), but ADHD, separation anxiety, and simple phobias were all diagnosed in more than 10% of the sample (Keenan, Shaw, Walsh, Delliquadri, & Giovannelli, 1997). In this same study, utilizing the CBCL, 18.2% of the children showed significant externalizing problems, and 9.6% had internalizing problems. When CBCL scores were used to predict DSM-III-R status, over 80% of the externalizing cases were correctly classified, whereas only 62% of the internalizing cases were correctly classified. Thus, although there is some overlap between the DSM and the CBCL, these methods do identify some children differently.

In a recent study of clinic-referred children, ages 2 to 5, the vast majority (about 80%) met criteria for at least one of the disruptive behavior disorders (ADHD, ODD, or CD), and many met criteria for two or three of these disorders (Keenan & Wakschlag, 2000). Thomas and Guskin (2001) found a slightly lower rate of disruptive behavior disorders in a sample of clinic-referred infants and preschoolers (ages 18–47 months): 34% met criteria for a disruptive behavior disorder, but the same percentage met criteria for an "emotional" disorder that included all of the internalizing disorders in the DSM-IV. However, it was noted that many children (45%) had significant levels of both internalizing and externalizing problems.

Although gender differences have not always been examined in prevalence studies, in general, boys are more likely than girls to exhibit externalizing behaviors in the preschool years and beyond. Both the type and the severity of problems exhibited by boys and girls in the early childhood years seem to be quite similar, although boys tend to exhibit more inappropriate physical behaviors (e.g., hitting) than girls (Webster-Stratton, 1996).

Given the lack of widespread agreement on how to diagnose young children with emotional or behavior problems, or even *whether* children should be diagnosed, the interpretation of the data from these prevalence studies is somewhat difficult. Differing prevalence rates likely have to do with differing applications of diagnostic criteria and different measures used in the diagnostic process. Many studies with young children simply identified children with high scores on behavior rating scales as those with significant problems. This method certainly has its advantages, and its application is becoming easier, given the growing number of rating scales that now have early childhood norms (see Chapter 2). However, DSM-IV diagnoses are also commonly used and are necessary in some situations (e.g., insurance reimbursement).

For the ease of communication, we have chosen to divide this book into general categories of disorders. Within each chapter we discuss specific DSM-IV disorders, when appropriate. However, it should be kept in mind that the interventions discussed in this text are not designed specifically for any one DSM disorder but, rather, are directed at treating the *specific set of symptoms* the child is exhibiting.

STABILITY OF BEHAVIOR PROBLEMS

An increasing body of literature has made it clear that behavior problems in preschool and kindergarten children are often (although not always) stable over time. Much of this research has focused on externalizing problems (e.g., conduct problems, general acting-out behaviors) and thus is most relevant to problems in this area. Considerably less is known regarding the stability of internalizing problems initially detected in preschool and kindergarten children. Of those children who are identified as having externalizing problems during the preschool years, approximately 50% will continue to have behavior problems over time (Campbell, 1995). These problems may persist not just over the preschool and early elementary school years, but into adolescence (McGee, Partridge, Williams, & Silva, 1991) and even adulthood (Huesmann, Eron, Lefkowitz, & Walder, 1984). The more severe the problems and the longer the problems have been present, the more likely the problems will continue to exist. For example, in a group of children initially classified as having "pervasive" externalizing problems during the preschool years, 94% were classified as having some form of externalizing problems in first grade. Similarly, children not classified as having behavior problems during the preschool years were unlikely to be classified as having problems in first grade (Heller, Baker, Henker, & Hinshaw, 1996).

Campbell and her colleagues have conducted numerous studies on preschool-age children and have followed many of these children over a number of years. In one group of children initially noted to have externalizing problems ("hard-to-manage") at age 3, approximately half continued to display such problems when evaluated at age 6 (Campbell, Ewing, Breaux, & Szumowski, 1986); of those who continued to have problems at age 6, approximately two-thirds met criteria for an externalizing disorder at age 9 (Campbell & Ewing, 1990). At age 13, these children were more likely to be diagnosed with ADHD or ODD/CD than control children not identified as having significant problems during the preschool years. At age 13, approximately half of the hard-to-manage children met criteria for ADHD (compared to 8% of the controls), and about 40% met criteria for ODD or CD (compared to 8% of the controls). Although the children initially classified as hard-to-manage were not more likely than the control children to meet criteria for an internalizing disorder, they were more likely to have co-occurring diagnoses (Pierce, Ewing, & Campbell, 1999).

A similar set of studies by Campbell and colleagues with boys found similar results. A large portion of boys initially identified as inattentive, overactive, or impulsive during the preschool years were rated as having continuing problems by parents (64%, according to maternal ratings; 47%, according to paternal ratings) or teachers (38%) at a 2-year follow-up (Campbell, 1994). At a follow-up at age 9, 34% of the hard-to-manage boys met criteria for ADHD, ODD, or CD, compared with only 13% of a control group. Boys who had persistent problems at age 6 were more likely to continue to have problems at age 9 than those whose problems improved at age 6 (59% vs. 24%). As with the other studies, the prevalence of internalizing disorders at age 9 was similar across boys in the hard-to-manage group and those in the control group (Pierce et al., 1999).

Given the findings from these studies, it seems likely that many children who are identified as having behavior problems during elementary school first exhibited symptoms of these problems during their preschool years. It is clear, then, that the preschool years are an ideal time to provide interventions for these problems. Although not all young children identified as having problems continue to have problems at later ages, certainly the substantial number of children who do continue to have problems warrants more attention to interventions for this age group. If interventions are successful with preschool- and kindergarten-age children, the number of children in need of interventions later in life and the complexity of the interventions needed should be dramatically reduced.

PREDICTORS OF PROBLEMS

With the mounting evidence that many preschool- and kindergarten-age children identified as having behavior problems continue to have such problems, researchers have turned to investigating the factors that mediate long-term outcomes. If (1) the factors that lead to initial and continued problems and (2) the factors that contribute to a decrease in later problems can be determined, then it would be easier to develop interventions and to target those interventions to the populations that would benefit the most from them. In the following sections (and in Tables 1.2 and 1.3), factors that have been noted to predict continuation of problems over time are summarized.

Predictors of Externalizing Problems

Many of the factors identified as contributing to both the initial expression of behavior problems as well as their long-term stability are related to characteristics of the child's family. Parenting behaviors are probably the most studied of these factors and have consistently been related to child behavior problems. Gerald Patterson is perhaps the best known for developing models in this area, and Patterson's coercive parenting cycle is cited extensively as a predictor of child externalizing problems (Patterson, 1982). Many of the family-based interventions for child behavior problems are based, in large part, on this

TABLE 1.2. Predictors of Externalizing Problems in Young Children

Parent characteristics	Child characteristics
Parenting behaviors (e.g., coercive parenting, negative discipline strategies)	Insecure attachment
	Difficult temperament
Parental stress	Initial severity of externalizing problems
Parental depression	
Low sense of parenting efficacy	Demographic variables
Family dysfunction	
Low social support	Lack of father involvement
	Low maternal age
	Low socioeconomic status

**TABLE 1.3. Predictors of Internalizing Problems
in Young Children**

Parent characteristics	Child characteristics
Parental stress	Difficult temperament
Parental conflict	Behaviorally inhibited temperament
	Insecure attachment
	Negative/noncompliant behaviors
	Initial severity of internalizing problems

model. In the coercive parenting pattern, parents make repeated requests of their children, who do not comply with the requests. Eventually the parent backs down from the request, due to the negative or aggressive behaviors exhibited by the child. Thus the parent negatively reinforces the child by withdrawing the aversive command or request. The parent, in turn, is negatively reinforced by the discontinuation of the aversive behaviors the child was exhibiting. Typically there is an escalation in this pattern, with parents eventually resorting to more severe methods of discipline in attempts to obtain compliance. The use of these severe methods is often reinforced by the child stopping his/her negative behaviors only once the severe methods are used. In this pattern, both the parent and child tend to escalate their use of negative and aggressive behaviors. Although Patterson's model of parenting was originally developed in relation to boys, research indicates that these same patterns also contribute to the development of antisocial behavior in girls (e.g., Eddy, Leve, & Fagot, 2001). These parenting patterns are likely present from early on in the parent–child relationship. In fact, studies with preschool children have demonstrated that low parental responsiveness and the use of harsh discipline increase the risk that preschool-age children will exhibit disruptive behaviors (Wakschlag & Keenan, 2001).

Parental stress   specifically, stress related to the parenting role also has been found to predict problem behaviors during the preschool years (Baker & Heller, 1996; Wakschlag & Keenan, 2001), as has a low sense of parenting efficacy (Baker & Heller, 1996). Additionally, maternal depression has been implicated as a potential risk factor. A recent study demonstrated that maternal depression alone did not negatively impact preschool-age children, but maternal depression that co-occurred with other problems did have a negative impact on later social–emotional development. This relationship was particularly strong for boys (Carter, Garrity-Rokous, Chazan-Cohen, Little, & Briggs-Gowan, 2001).

Parental stress and family dysfunction are important in predicting both the initial onset of problems as well as the continuation of such problems. In their longitudinal work in this area, Campbell and her colleagues (Campbell, Pierce, Moore, Marakovitz, & Newby, 1996) noted that boys identified during their preschool years as being hard-to-manage were most likely to continue to have problems through age 9 if their mothers reported experiencing high levels of stress and if the mother–child relationship was particularly problematic. Those preschoolers who experienced less family stress began to improve by early elementary school. Interestingly, in a comparison group of children (i.e., those not identified as having problems during the preschool years), the boys were more likely to have externalizing problems at age 9 if mothers reported high levels of stress, and mothers reporting high levels of stress were more likely to use negative discipline strategies than mothers reporting low levels of stress. Thus Campbell and her colleagues note the importance of family stress and negative discipline in relationship to child externalizing problems over time.

Although much of the research on behavior problems in preschool children has focused on parent characteristics, more recently the research focus has turned to both child and parent characteristics and the link between the two. Studies examining predictors of problems in the preschool years, as well as the continuation of such problems, have identified both parent and child characteristics that contribute to this process. Attachment is one specific child variable that has been examined. Children with insecure attachments have been found to be more at risk for later behavior problems. This risk is particularly applicable to children who have a disorganized type of attachment, but other types of insecure attachments may also lead to long-term problems, most notably when combined with other risk factors (Shaw, Owens, Vondra, Keenan, & Winslow, 1996).

Demographic variables also have been related to preschool and kindergarten behavior problems. For example, lack of father involvement has been associated with ADHD, and low maternal age at the time of the child's birth has been associated with CD (Keenan & Wakschlag, 2000). Socioeconomic status (SES) also has been linked to behavior problems, with children from lower-SES families typically exhibiting more problem behaviors than those from higher-SES families (Campbell, 1995). Biological factors such as low birth weight also may play a role in the development of problem behaviors, although research in this area is not consistent (Campbell, 1995).

As noted earlier, a consistent predictor of behavior problem stability over time is the initial severity of such problems. Numerous studies (e.g., Campbell, 1987; Campbell & Ewing, 1990; Pierce et al., 1999) have shown that children who initially have more problems and problems of greater intensity are less likely to experience a decline in behavior problems than children with fewer and/or less severe initial problems.

Although much of the research on predictors of behavior problems during the preschool and kindergarten years has focused on problem behaviors in general (rather than specific diagnostic categories), a recent study (Shaw, Owens, Giovannelli, & Winslow, 2001) examined differential predictors for the three externalizing disorders (ADHD, ODD, and CD), as diagnosed at age 6. Results indicated that children with comorbid disorders had more difficult temperaments and more behavior problems during infancy. In addition, mothers of these children had higher rates of depression and aggression, less social support, and more rejecting parenting styles. Children with CD only tended to show more problems early on and have difficult temperaments, but few other factors were predictive of problems. In contrast, children diagnosed only with ODD tended to have less difficult temperaments and had not exhibited problem behaviors from early on. Instead, their parents tended to be rejecting, and mothers tended to have high levels of depression and aggression. Children in the ADHD group were similar to nonproblem children in terms of risk factors.

Predictors of Internalizing Problems

Although researchers are beginning to develop a clearer picture of what leads to externalizing disorders in young children, and which factors related to young children and their families predict these disorders later in life, the profile for internalizing disorders in the preschool years is much less clear. Studies that have examined factors in this area have had similar findings to studies that examined predictors of externalizing problems. For example, a difficult temperament, negative and noncompliant behaviors, and higher levels of internalizing problems during the preschool years, as well as high maternal stress, have been implicated as early predictors of later internalizing problems (Campbell & Ewing, 1990). In a study that examined predictors of both internalizing and externalizing symptoms, it was found that early aggression and noncompliance were related to externalizing problems in later preschool years, whereas a difficult temperament was more likely to lead to internalizing problems (Keenan, Shaw, Delliquadri, Giovannelli, & Walsh, 1998).

In a study examining the predictors of internalizing disorders more specifically (Shaw, Keenan, Vondra, Delliquadri, & Giovannelli, 1997), young children were more likely to be rated as having internalizing problems if they displayed "negative emotionality," had a disorganized attachment, and had parents who had a high level of negative life change experiences, had high exposure to parental conflict. The first two variables at age 2 or under, as well internalizing symptoms at age 3, predicted the presence of internalizing symptoms at age 5. For both withdrawal and anxiety/depression, there was a significant interaction between infant difficulty (negative emotionality) and conflict exposure, suggesting that children who are difficult may be at increased risk of experiencing negative reactions to conflict exposure.

With regard to specific internalizing disorders, researchers have examined the connection between (1) later anxiety disorders and (2) the early childhood characteristics of temperament and parent–child attachment in some detail. Both of these variables have been linked to later anxiety disorders. Preschool-age children who are more fearful and shy, as well as those who have an insecure attachment to a caregiver, are more at risk for receiving a later diagnosis of an anxiety disorder (Bernstein, Borchardt, & Perwien, 1996).

Infant temperament styles also have been linked to later anxiety disorders. In several studies, researchers identified children in the preschool years who were "behaviorally inhibited" and followed these children for a number of years. In one such study, children identified as being inhibited prior to age 3 were more likely to have a social anxiety disorder in adolescence (Schwartz, Snidman, & Kagan, 1999). Other work has indicated higher prevalence rates for a number of anxiety disorders for children identified as having a behaviorally inhibited temperament (Biederman, Rosenbaum, Chaloff, & Kagan, 1995).

Insecure attachment of the anxious/resistant type was found to be related to later anxiety disorders in a group of children initially evaluated at age 1. When these children were evaluated as adolescents, those who had shown an anxious/resistant attachment at age 1 were more likely to receive an anxiety disorder diagnosis than were other children their age. This type of attachment predicted anxiety, even after taking into account the relationship between child anxiety and maternal anxiety and the relationship between anxiety and temperament (Warren, Huston, Egeland, & Sroufe, 1997).

CHAPTER SUMMARY/PURPOSE OF BOOK

Social and emotional problems during the early childhood years are clearly a real problem with potentially adverse long-term outcomes. Given that problems identified during the preschool and kindergarten years often do continue, it is imperative that treatments be provided for these children and their families to prevent negative outcomes. Although research on the treatment of early childhood mental health problems is still in the beginning stages, a number of psychosocial treatments have been validated for use with preschool children or show particular promise for use with this age group. The purpose of this book is to provide a review of, and implementation guidelines for, these psychosocial interventions. Clinicians should be able to use the information and materials provided in this book to develop treatment plans for most of the disorders commonly seen during the preschool and kindergarten years.

2

Assessment of Mental Health Issues in Preschool and Kindergarten Children

The assessment of emotional and behavioral problems in preschool- and kindergarten-age children has become an increasingly important task over the past few decades. Within the field of mental health, a greater emphasis has been placed on early identification and intervention for young children with emotional and behavioral problems. Mental health professionals have realized that by the time a child reaches school age, he/she may have missed vital interventions that could have thwarted later, more serious problems. Changes beginning just a decade ago pushed the concept of early intervention into the forefront of social policy (Shonkoff & Meisels, 1990). In order for early intervention to occur, there must be assessment measures that can adequately and accurately identify young children with mental health problems and other special needs. Unfortunately, many challenges remain when attempting to assess and diagnose young children. These challenges range from a general lack of assessment measures designed specifically for this population, to problems with the technical adequacy of those social–emotional assessment instruments that *are* available for use with young children. In addition, the social and emotional behavior of young children is often variable and can be influenced by contexts and settings, which can make it difficult to obtain reliable behavior ratings (Merrell, 1999).

Though challenges still exist in the assessment of young children, encouraging developments have emerged over the last decade. An increasing number of behavior rating scales, designed specifically for the assessment of preschool- and kindergarten-age children, have become available. In addition, as research on observations and interviews of preschool- and kindergarten-age children has increased, historic beliefs that useful information could not be obtained from young children have been challenged and revised. This chapter provides an overview of these measures and techniques, highlighting those that have the best reliability and validity for preschool and kindergarten populations. A word of caution is necessary: Though these techniques and measures are, in general, "user friendly," and teachers, parents, and other professionals can be trained to conduct observations, it is recommended that a mental health professional with appropriate background and training, such as a school psychologist or child clinical psychologist, administer and interpret any measures used, and that only a skilled clinician conduct clinical interviews.

INTERVIEWS WITH PARENTS AND TEACHERS

Parent and teacher/daycare worker interviews are crucial to gaining a comprehensive understanding of the young child. The chief complaint and referral for services almost always comes from adults in the child's life, such as parents or teachers. Therefore, an important element in the assessment of the young child is to clarify who has concerns about the child and what specifically these concerns are. Conducting an interview with key adults is the primary way of gathering this information.

Parent/Caregiver Interviews

The parents' or guardians' consent, cooperation, and participation are critical in the assessment of young children*. The parent is often the best source of information regarding the child's history, current difficulties, and outside factors that may be impacting the child's behavior, such as family problems, a death in the family, or a recent move. In addition, the parent is an invaluable resource for connecting the clinician with other key adults in the child's life, so that the interviewer can gather as much information as possible about the child. The parent can also provide the clinician with the necessary consents so that he/she can consent with other providers. An example of a consent form is provided in Figure 2.1.

The first task in the parent interview is to build rapport. One way to help put the parent at ease is to introduce yourself, shake the parent's hand, and discuss the purpose of the interview and assessment. Any questions the parent has about the assessment process should also be answered. It is important to empower parents by letting them know you are there to help them and their child, and that they are crucial to the process because they are the "experts" on their child. This straightforward approach demystifies the assessment process and helps ensure the parents' cooperation during the interview and evaluation sessions.

During the interview the clinician gathers information about the referral question or presenting problem behaviors. The frequency, intensity, duration, and circumstances in which the problem behaviors occur, and the perceptions of the adults, child, and others about the behaviors, are important to ascertain (American Academy of Child and Adolescent Psychiatry, 1997b). It is common for parents, caregivers, and other adults in the child's life to differ in how they perceive the problem behavior. For example, one parent

---

*To simplify wording throughout this text, we refer primarily to parents, with the understanding that this usage also includes nonparent caregivers.

CONSENT TO OBTAIN OR RELASE CONFIDENTIAL INFORMATION

Identifying Client Information

Name: _____ Date: _____

AKA, if any: _____ Date of birth: _____

Client ID number: _____

I hereby authorize and request the exchange of information and/or release of psychiatric and/or medical treatment and/or school records accumulated during the period beginning (month/day/year)_____ through (month/day/year) _____ between:

Name of Releasing Individual, Title: _____

Agency, Address, City, State, Zip: _____

_____

<u>and</u>

Name of Requesting Individual, Title: _____

Agency, Address, City, State, Zip: _____

_____

For the purpose of:

    Evaluation _____   Treatment Planning _____   Other (specify) _____

Information to be released/exchanged (specify):

_____

_____

_____

_____

This consent can be revoked by the undersigned grantor at any time. If not revoked earlier, it shall terminate at the end of: _____ 3 months _____ 6 months _____ 12 months

Parent or Guardian Signature: _____ Date: _____

Witness Signature: _____ Date: _____

Professional Signature: _____ Date: _____

Date release mailed: _____ Date materials mailed: _____

FIGURE 2.1. Example of a written release of information form. From Gretchen A. Gimpel and Melissa L. Holland (2003). Copyright by The Guilford Press. Permission to photocopy this figure is granted to purchasers of this book for personal use only (see copyright page for details).

may see the behavior as being extremely problematic, whereas the other may not see the behavior as a problem at all. These differences may be related to a variety of factors, including the amount of time the adult spends with the child, the circumstances surrounding the time spent with the child, the ideas each adult has about developmentally appropriate childhood behaviors, and how each adult interacts with the child. It is up to the interviewer to determine the factors involved in these differences by conducting careful interviews with all key adults in the child's life and through observations of the child. In addition, children often exhibit different behaviors in different settings, depending on the expectations in each setting. For example, a child with few structured activities or demands at home may not exhibit many problem behaviors with his/her parents, whereas in the structured preschool setting, the child may have difficulty staying seated or attending to the teacher. Here, too, it is up to the interviewer to sort through the factors involved in each setting to obtain a full diagnostic picture of the child.

In addition to identifying specific problem behaviors, one primary purpose for interviewing parents is to obtain a report of relevant background information on the child (Merrell, 1999). Background and developmental information is necessary to provide a detailed history of the child's physical and cognitive development, as well as his/her social, emotional, and behavioral history and development. Even if the parents are unable to provide the interviewer with a detailed developmental history (as often is the case when working with foster parents), they can still provide a meaningful account of the child's relationship with others or important events that may have helped shape the child's development (American Academy of Child and Adolescent Psychiatry, 1997b). Core elements to be included in an interview with parents are discussed in the following material (American Academy of Child and Adolescent Psychiatry, 1997b; Merrell, 1999; Sattler, 1998). A summary of these areas is provided in Table 2.1 and an example of an intake interview (which would be used by the clinician to structure the interview) is included in Figure 2.2.

Family Relationships

How the child relates to family members, including parents, siblings, and extended family, should be covered in the interview. Changes within the family system, such as birth of siblings, deaths, divorce, removal from the home, and changes in caretaking arrangements, such as custody and visitation, also should be noted. In addition, it is important to inquire about the child's compliance with family rules and parental disciplinary practices.

TABLE 2.1. Areas for Inclusion in a Clinical Interview with Parents or Caregivers

Family relationships	Emotional development and temperament
Cognitive and school functioning	Interests and talents
Peer relationships	Strengths
Physical development	Unusual circumstances
Child medical and psychiatric history	Prior testing
Family medical and psychiatric history	

CHILD INTAKE

I. General Background

Child's name: _____

Age: _____ Date of birth: _____ Sex: _____ Grade: _____

Who is at home?

Mother: _____ Natural Foster Step Adoptive

Father: _____ Natural Foster Step Adoptive

Other children:

Name	Age	Sex	Grade	Relation

Other adults:

Name	Relationship to child

Parents' marital status:

If separated: Name of other parent: _____

Involvement with child: _____

Who referred you? _____

Reason for referral: _____

_____

II. Parent and Other Children Assessment

Education—Highest level completed:

Mother _____ Father _____

Current employment:

Mother _____

Father _____

Home schedule of:

Mother _____

Father _____

(continued)

FIGURE 2.2. Intake Interview. From Gretchen A. Gimpel and Melissa L. Holland (2003). Copyright by The Guilford Press. Permission to photocopy this figure is granted to purchasers of this book for personal use only (see copyright page for details).

Has either parent ever received therapy?   Yes _____   No _____

    If yes, describe: _____

_____

_____

Level of marital satisfaction during past month: _____

Level of marital satisfaction during past 6 months: _____

Do any of your other children have emotional or behavioral problems of concern?

    Yes _____   No _____

    If yes, describe: _____

_____

_____

III. Child Medical and Developmental History

Complications during pregnancy?   Yes _____   No _____

    If yes, describe: _____

_____

Complications during delivery?   Yes _____   No _____

    If yes, describe: _____

_____

At what age did child first:

    Sit alone _____   Crawl _____   Walk _____

    Talk (one word) _____   Talk (sentences) _____

Does the child have any current health problems?   Yes _____   No _____

    If yes, what? _____

_____

Is the child currently on any medications?   Yes _____   No _____

    If yes: Medication and dose: _____

                For what was it prescribed? _____

                How long has child been on it? _____

                Who prescribed it? _____

                How does it affect behavior? _____

Any past medications: _____

_____

Any hospitalizations?   Yes _____   No _____

    If yes, list: _____

(continued)

Any ER episodes? Yes _____ No _____

    If yes, list: _____

Any significant illnesses? Yes _____ No _____

    If yes, list: _____

How is current health? _____

Any problems with:

    Vision _____ Hearing _____ Speech _____

Any medical conditions that run in the family (e.g., diabetes, thyroid problems, cancer)?

    Yes _____ No _____

    If yes, describe: _____

IV. Child Behavioral/Emotional Assessment

Has child received mental health services before? Yes _____ No _____

    If yes, describe: _____

_____

_____

Describe a typical day for your child:

_____

_____

_____

_____

What time does your child typically go to bed? _____ And wake up? _____

Has your child experienced any traumatic events? Yes _____ No _____

    If yes, what and when: _____

Has anyone else in family had problems similar to those of the child?

    Yes _____ No _____

    If yes, please describe: _____

Are there any psychiatric conditions that run in the family (e.g., depression, ADHD)?

    Yes _____ No _____

    If yes, please describe: _____

How is child's relationship with:

    Mother _____

    Father _____

How does child get along with peers? _____

Describe child's friendships: _____

How does child get along with siblings? _____

(continued)

25

V. Academic and Social History

Current school: _____   Teacher: _____

Past schools attended: _____

Teacher reports of academic progress: _____

Special Education placement? _____

Other help: _____

Behavioral problems in school: _____

_____

VI. Assessment of Behavior Management

Who ordinarily disciplines child? _____

How is child disciplined? _____

_____

How often is child disciplined? _____

Which form of discipline is most effective? _____

_____

What disciplinary approaches have been tried that have *not* worked? _____

_____

Do parents agree on reasons for and types of discipline? _____

VII. Current Concerns

What are your top three concerns at this time?

_____

_____

_____

Name three things you think your child does well.

_____

_____

_____

Cognitive and School Functioning

The parents' understanding of the child's cognitive strengths and weaknesses, along with academic progress and school/daycare functioning, should be addressed. Areas to be explored include the child's ability to separate from the parent to attend school or daycare; the child's verbal, attentional, and organizational skills; the child's motivation to learn (if in a school setting); and the child's relationships with staff and teachers. If records of past school-related services (e.g., early intervention programs) are available, the interviewer should request copies from the parent or obtain consent from the parent to contact the appropriate organization for these records.

Peer Relationships

The interviewer should inquire about the child's friendships with other children his/her age in the daycare, school, church, or neighborhood settings. Social skills and deficits should be explored.

Development

The child's developmental history, including prenatal care, pregnancy/birth complications, and developmental milestone achievement, are critical pieces of information to explore with the parent. Important questions to ask include:

- Was the child was exposed prenatally to alcohol, illicit substances, or medications?
- Was the child premature?
- Were there any complications during pregnancy or birth?
- Did the child require an extended hospital stay after birth?

The interviewer also should inquire about developmental milestone achievement, such as ages at which the child walked and talked.

Child and Family Medical and Psychiatric History

Medical and psychiatric history of the child and his/her family of origin can provide information relevant to the current presentation of the child. Inquiries about hospitalizations, allergies, health problems, sensory problems (such as vision or hearing loss), injuries (including head injuries), and operations, as well as the child's reactions to these illnesses and events, can provide important developmental information about the child. The interviewer also should obtain any psychiatric records that may exist for the child, including reports from previous evaluations and/or therapy sessions. In addition, family medical and psychiatric history should be explored to help determine if there is a familial pattern of any problems.

Emotional Development and Temperament

This category includes information about the child's personality, style of attachment to caregivers, temperament, present and past mood regulation, and adaptability to novel or difficult situations. The assessment of mood should cover past and current presence of depressive, anxious, and other psychologically relevant symptoms.

Interests, Talents, and Strengths

In addition to obtaining information about the problem behaviors the child is exhibiting, the interviewer also should inquire about the child's areas of strengths and talents. Important areas to cover include what the child likes to do for fun at home and school, if the child is especially proficient in a particular developmental area, and the parents' perceptions of the child's strengths.

Traumatic Circumstances

Unusual or traumatic circumstances include events such as child physical abuse, sexual abuse, neglect, family violence, natural disasters, or other exposure to other traumatic events. The interviewer should determine if any such events occurred and, if so, the impact of the exposure should be explored, along with reviewing any Child Protective Service records or medical records, which could be helpful in piecing together information about the severity and effects of the situation on the child.

Prior Testing

As previously mentioned, any past psychological testing should be obtained in order to aid the interviewer in the present assessment of the child. For example, some children have had developmental assessments conducted when toddlers, or screening assessments administered when entering preschool, such as Head Start. These pieces of information can be useful in determining prior functioning and the young child's foundational skills.

Teacher/Daycare Worker Interviews

Teachers, daycare workers, and other important adults in the child's life can provide a wealth of information about the child outside of the home setting. The teacher/daycare provider interview is conducted somewhat differently from the interview with the parent, in that the teacher/daycare provider likely will not have much background information or developmental information on the child. Instead information from these sources would relate to the child's relations with peers and adults, the child's mastery of beginning key concepts/academic skills, and the child's ability to meet expectations of the school or daycare setting.

During the interview, it is important to build rapport and gain the cooperation of the teacher/daycare worker in order to gain as much information regarding the child's problems and strengths as possible. Prior to conducting this interview, the clinician should ensure he/she has a signed release-of-information form from the parent (see Figure 2.1). The teacher/daycare worker should be approached from a team standpoint, as someone whom you believe can help remediate existing problems in the school/daycare setting and facilitate the child's experience of success. Once the assessment has been completed, it is important to share any recommendations for interventions that relate specifically to the school or daycare environment with the teacher/daycare provider. If necessary, the teacher/daycare provider should be made aware of other professionals who can help him/her implement the necessary interventions, such as a behavioral specialist, school psychologist, or the child's individual therapist.

INTERVIEWS WITH YOUNG CHILDREN

A variety of theories and thoughts regarding the usefulness of interviewing young children have been expressed over the years. The saying "children should be seen, not heard" reflects a common adult perception that children do not have anything useful or important to say. Young children, in particular, are often viewed as illogical and unable to distinguish reality from fantasy. The work of developmental theorists added some support to these beliefs. For example, in Piaget's theory of cognitive development, it is assumed that, although children between the ages of 2 and 7 are able to represent thoughts with words, they lack the ability to engage in logical reasoning (Piaget, 1983). Theories such as this have led some to believe that important information cannot be reliably obtained from young children. Although the type of information one can obtain from young children in an interview is limited, it is possible to obtain salient information about children's feelings, interests, and concerns (Sattler, 1998). However, because of the limitations associated with interviewing young children, it is recommended that any information obtained from a young child via an interview be combined with other relevant information, such as parent and teacher interviews, rating scale data, and clinical judgment, to achieve the fullest possible clinical picture of the young child.

When interviewing a young child, it is important to keep in mind key developmental issues. Young children are often shy and timid in initial interview situations and likely will have difficulty verbalizing thoughts and feelings (Sattler, 1998). Preschoolers typically define others in concrete, inflexible terms, such as thinking someone is all good or all bad, without the understanding that the person can exhibit both qualities (Keith & Campbell, 2000; Sattler, 1998). In addition, because preschool- and kindergarten-age children are typically unable to sustain attention on any one task for a long period of time, they may need to be interviewed over several sessions. Seeing a child multiple times also can prove beneficial for rapport building. Young children are typically more active and impulsive than the older children, creating, at times, a challenging situation for the interviewer. Redirection is often helpful to refocus the child, as is simply saying the child's name frequently during the conversation. Giving the child frequent reinforcers (such as stickers or candy) for staying on task also can be helpful. However, it is important that the child does not perceive that he/she is being rewarded for a certain type of answer. Such an impression could influence the child to change his/her response set (e.g., when the interviewer asks about fears, the child says that he/she is afraid of school when he/she actually likes school). It also can be helpful to use statements such as "Let's put our ears on for these questions," or, to validate the child's feelings about the questions, "I know this question might be hard to answer, but I need you to think about it and give me an answer." These statements can help the child focus and respond to the interviewer's inquiries. Finally, young children have limited verbal capabilities, making it necessary for the interviewer to pay attention to other aspects of the child's presentation along with the child's words. The clinician should attend to the child's depth and style of personal relatedness, mood, gestures, themes covered in play or conversation, range of emotions expressed, and contact with the clinician (Greenspan & Greenspan, 1991).

Despite the difficulties of interviewing young children, such interviews can provide valuable information that may not be available from other sources: such as the level of the child's suffering, any thought distortions that may exist, anxious and depressed symptoms, and "secrets" that are detrimental for the child to keep. The interviewer therefore must be attuned to what the young child is expressing in the interview setting as well as to the factors which may be impacting the quality of the information obtained. In addition to the limited cognitive capacity of preschool- and kindergarten-age children, factors such as the level of rapport established, the context of the interview, and the motivation of the child are important in determining the validity of the interview. The mental status of the child also should be noted during the interview process.

Rapport Building/Initial Information Gathering

Rapport between the young child and the interviewer is established somewhat differently than the rapport-building process used with older children or adults—though it is just as, if not more, important to establish. The initial step in any interview with a young child is to put him/her at ease. The young child may have difficulty separating from his/her parents. If this difficulty occurs, the best practice is to invite the parent and child into the office together, so that the child will feel more comfortable with the situation and setting. It is often helpful to give the child the opportunity to engage in a nonthreatening activity, such as coloring or playing with a toy. Once the child begins to feel comfortable in the surroundings, the interviewer can ask the parents, in a matter-of-fact manner, to go into the other room (Merrell, 1999). Most likely, this sequence will be all that is needed for the child to feel comfortable with the process. If the child becomes upset, reassure him/her that the parent is right outside the office and that he/she will be able to see his/her mom or dad when finished. Obviously, if the child becomes extremely upset, the interview may need to be discontinued and rescheduled for another time.

Once the child is in the office, the first step to a successful interview is to gain the child's attention by engaging him/her. Interviewers at times make the mistake of attempting to get an inattentive child to verbalize before the child is fully attending to the interviewer and the situation (Greenspan & Greenspan, 1991). In addition to gaining the child's attention, the interviewer must also build rapport with him/her. Typically this is done through child-directed play activities. The clinician should have available toys appropriate to the child's developmental level as well as toys that will facilitate communication. Drawing materials, dolls, play-dough, clay, or other nondisruptive manipulatives can be useful for engaging the child in an acceptable and nonthreatening activity. When building rapport, the clinician should focus on describing the child's activities as well as reflecting verbalizations (which may be minimal) and refrain from probing too much for information.

Drawing techniques also may be used to help build rapport as well as to gather information. The kinetic family drawing, in which the child draws a picture of him/herself and family doing something together, or the self-portrait, in which the child draws a picture of him/herself, can provide a way for the young child to express feelings and concerns through a developmentally appropriate mode of communication while also helping the child feel more comfortable and engaged. In addition, these drawings can provide the interviewer with helpful information, such as (1) the presence of any notable developmental delays in fine motor skills, (2) who the child includes in his/her family drawing, (3) how the child perceives him/herself, and (4) the presence of any abuse themes, such as people drawn without clothing, with genitalia, etc. Although formal scoring systems (Koppitz, 1968) are available for each of these drawing activities, it is not recommended that they be used as formal assessment measures due to their poor psychometric properties (Chandler & Johnson, 1991).

Once the clinician begins to ask questions, other play-based methods also can be helpful in facilitating the interview process. For example, puppets can be quite useful when asking children questions that may feel threatening to them. For example, the examiner can ask the child's puppet the questions, request that the puppet "find out" the answer from the child and allow the puppet to respond. To aid in determining the validity of the responses, the examiner can ask the puppet several nonthreatening questions about the child, to which the examiner can validate the answers (e.g., the child's hair color or name).

In cases of suspected physical or sexual abuse, the use of anatomically correct dolls can help the child demonstrate what happened while keeping his/her focus on the doll rather than self, which may prove to be too overwhelming for the child. However, children between the ages of 3 and 5 may not need many toys during the interview if the purpose is to investigate acknowledged or alleged abuse (Sattler, 1998).

Finally, story-telling techniques, such as asking the child to make up stories in response to neutral pictures, drawings, or doodles, can encourage the child to deal with information or feelings that may cause shame, fear, or guilt, while providing the interviewer with themes about what may have happened to the child (Brooks, 1985; Garbarino et al., 1992).

In addition to the use of play during the interview with the child, a free-play session can be helpful for the interviewer to gain more insight into the young child's world. Suggested play materials for use during a free-play session (Axline, 1969) are listed in Table 2.2. Sattler (1998) offers observational guidelines to use when observing preschoolers in a free-play setting. These guidelines include observing the following indicators:

- How the child enters the playroom
- How the child initiates play

TABLE 2.2. Suggested Play Materials for Free-Play Session

Doll family	Clay
Dollhouse	Finger paints
Doll furniture	Toy telephone
Nursing bottles	Toy cars and airplanes
Toy soldiers	Newspaper and magazine pictures
Sandbox	Construction paper
Toy animals	Crayons
Baby dolls	Toy dishes
Puppets	

Source. Axline (1969).

- How much energy the child puts into the play
- What verbalizations and body movements the child makes
- The child's affect during the play
- The tone and integration of the play
- The child's content of play and creativity
- The child's preference in play objects
- How the child interacts with the adult in the play
- The child's departure from the playroom

The interviewer's observations may provide important information about (1) the child's ability to adapt to new situations, (2) his/her thoughts and fantasies, (3) his/her ability to solve problems, (4) his/her degree of spontaneity and creativity, and (5) any interpersonal problems and the quality of interpersonal interactions (Sattler, 1998).

Context of the Interview

As mentioned previously, young children's behaviors can vary widely across time and settings, making it difficult to accurately perceive what the young child may be experiencing. Therefore, the context of the interview must be taken into account. Garbarino et al. (1992) discuss context in two categories. The first category includes *contexts relevant to the immediate assessment situation,* such as the social interaction between the child and adult, the physical setting, and the meaning of the event to the child. The second category includes *background contexts,* such as the child's familial, educational, and cultural history, as well as broader contexts of law and custom. Both categories can affect the young child's willingness to communicate.

In the first category, the immediate assessment situation, many factors can affect the way in which a young child responds to the interviewer. For example, the child may respond differently if he/she knows the interviewer than if the interviewer is a stranger. Because young children are often shy and timid in new settings (Sattler, 1998), it is likely the young child would be apprehensive initially with the unknown person, taking a longer time to establish rapport. With an interviewer the child knows, the child may answer the questions according to what the child thinks the interviewer would want to hear, based on past experience with that person.

The way the interviewer asks questions of the young child also can have a significant impact on what type of information is obtained. If leading or closed-ended questions are used, it is likely that the young child will respond in the way in which he/she thinks the interviewer would like, thereby potentially giving inaccurate or false reports of what happened. This pitfall is particularly likely with preschool-age children, who are more inclined to please adults than are older children (Hughes & Baker, 1990). Note the difference between the following two examples:

Leading (closed-ended) question: "Your mommy hits you, right?"
Nonleading (open-ended) question: "What does your mommy do when she gets mad at you?"

Clinicians should avoid asking too many questions, instead using descriptive statements for much of the interview. For example, rather than saying, "What are you drawing in that picture?" the clinician might say, "That's a nice picture. It looks like some children playing." However, it can be difficult to obtain information from a preschool-age child simply through the use of nonquestioning statements such as "Tell me about your friends." Thus it is recommended that a combination of short, probing (but nonleading) questions designed to clarify statements, open-ended questions, and statements designed to encourage the child to talk (e.g., "Ummm," "I see") be used with preschool-age children (Hughes & Baker, 1990; Sattler, 1998).

Stating what the child is doing in his/her play behaviors also can open up relevant conversation (e.g., if the dolls are hitting one another, state, "Wow, that mommy is sure mad at her babies. Some mommies do get that mad. What does your mommy do when she gets that mad?"). Note that young children, due to their limited vocabulary and cognitive abilities, are more apt to act out difficult feelings and situations than to verbalize how they are feeling.

Another factor that may affect the way a child responds is the setting in which the interview is conducted. The young child may respond differently if he/she is in a hospital or police station than a place in which the child feels comfortable and safe. The interviewer may not be able to change some of these factors, but it is important to recognize the potential impact of the factors on the child.

In addition, the perceived outcome of the interview may influence a child's motivation to participate or the responses the child provides. For example, the abused child who has been threatened with harm by a parent if he/she talks about the abuse would likely be motivated either to not talk to the interviewer or to deny that any abuse has occurred. With preschool- and kindergarten-age children, this situation can be very difficult. The use of rapport-building techniques, combined with simple reassurance and keen observation, is necessary to gather information in these cases. If the child gives any leads, such as "My daddy is mean," it is best to restate the phrase into a question, "Your daddy is mean?" and then ask more about this statement, such as, "Tell me how your daddy is mean" (Sattler, 1998).

The second context category includes broader issues related to culture, educational and familial history, and laws and customs (Garbarino et al., 1992). Cultural differences between the interviewer and the child can impact the process in several ways. First, cultural differences may be misinterpreted as pathology or as disrespect. For example, in some Native American cultures it is considered disrespectful to engage in direct eye contact (Sue & Sue, 1990), whereas in the mainstream American culture, absence of eye contact could indicate a lack of respect or that the person is lying or anxious. These culturally based differences must be investigated further if they do arise, so that the child is not needlessly pathologized. Consulting with a person from the same cultural background of the child can help the interviewer obtain further information about that culture and its associated practices.

Another form of cultural influence that can affect the interview process occurs when children have assimilated, through contact with parents or community, a general "cultural mistrust" of persons not of their culture. The child who is not trusting of outsiders may give only limited information in an interview or may lie to protect family members. It could be helpful to interview the child's parents or other family members to gain a better understanding of the familial beliefs before talking with the child. Children from families who have frequent negative contact with law enforcement or social service agencies may have learned to be distrustful and to not share information with others.

Finally, laws and customs also may have an impact on what information is obtained from a child. For example, some children may believe that they will be punished for speaking out. A generalization that examiners must avoid when interviewing children is that "children always tell the truth because they don't know how to lie." Obviously this is a dangerous misassumption; as discussed earlier, children's motivations during the interview process are highly salient and must be taken into account.

Mental Status Examination

The mental status examination (MSE), which combines information obtained from the interview as well as from informal observation of the child, can provide critical pieces of information about a child that aid in assessment, diagnosis, and intervention. For example, the MSE can reveal whether the child (1) appears to be physically neglected or abused (e.g., underweight, unkempt, dirty appearance, scars, marks or bruises), (2) is behind developmentally or cognitively (e.g., unable to complete tasks his/her peers can perform), or (3) appears especially anxious (e.g., fidgeting, frightened, or emotionally labile). The key elements in a general MSE often include the following: orientation to time, place, and person; physical appearance; affect and mood; speech and language; cognition, including thought content and estimated level of intelligence; insight and judgment; and perception, such as problems with hallucinations or delusions (American Academy of Child and Adolescent Psychiatry, 1997b). Obviously these areas must be adapted to the young child's presentation. For example, many young children may not know where they are, what day or time it is, or have adequate vocabulary or maturity to identify feeling states. Perceptual problems would most likely be present only if the young child were delirious due to a medical problem, environmental condition (such as fumes), or a medication/substance. It also would be important to differentiate between fantasy (in which preschool- and kindergarten-age children often engage) and a perceptual problem. The clinician could ask follow-up questions to help determine which is occurring. In general, clinicians should use their common sense and have a good understanding of developmental stages when observing, interviewing, and determining the mental status of a young child.

RATING SCALES

Rating scales, which require parents and/or teachers to indicate how often a child performs a variety of behaviors, have several advantages over other types of assessment procedures, particularly for young children: (1) Rating scales permit the collection and quantification of data regarding the occurrence of infrequent behaviors likely to be missed by observations (Barkley, 1998); (2) they can be used to gather information from different individuals who are responsible for the care and management of the child in different settings (Blondis, Snow, Stein, & Roizen, 1991); (3) they usually have normative data available to establish the statistical significance of the child's behavior (Guevremont, DuPaul & Barkley, 1993); and (4) they are relatively inexpensive and easy to administer (Ross & Ross, 1982). Particularly with young children, rating scales can provide reliable and valid diagnostic data, whereas other procedures, such as child interviews, may not.

Although rating scales have a number of advantages that make them particularly well-suited for use with kindergarten- and preschool-age children, it was not until relatively recently that researchers and clinicians started developing and norming rating scales specifically for use with younger children. Over the past decade, or so, rating scales for this population have increased in number. Most of these scales have involved downward extensions of existing scales (e.g., the preschool versions of the Child Behavior Checklist), although some were developed specifically for this population (e.g., the Preschool and Kindergarten Behavior Scale). This section provides an overview of psychometrically sound behavior rating scales designed for use with the preschool and kindergarten population.

Child Behavior Checklist and Teacher's Report Form

The Child Behavior Checklist (CBCL; Achenbach, 1991a) is a widely used measure for the assessment of problem behaviors in children. This scale and its school-version counterpart, the Teacher's Report Form (TRF; Achenbach, 1991b), are often used as screeners to determine areas in which children are exhibiting problem behaviors. Normative data are available for children ages 4–18 on the CBCL and for ages 5–18 years on the TRF. Recently revised versions of this scale now cover ages 6–18 for both the parent and teacher versions (Achenbach & Rescorla, 2001). The CBCL and TRF are among the most widely used rating scales designed for parents and caregivers to assess problem behaviors of children. These scales have been found to be psychometrically sound, with good reliability and validity (Achenbach, 1991a, 1991b).

Downward extensions of the CBCL and TRF have been developed specifically for preschool-age children. These include the Child Behavior Checklist for Ages 2–3 (CBCL 2–3; Achenbach, 1992) and the Caregiver–Teacher Report Form for Ages 2–5 (C-TRF 2–5; Achenbach, 1997), which have recently been revised as the CBCL 1½–5 and the C-TRF 1½–5 (Achenbach & Rescorla, 2000). The CBCL 1½–5 (normed on 700 children) and C-TRF 1½–5 (normed on 1,192 children) both have 99 items that are geared more specifically to reflect problem behaviors toddlers and preschoolers tend to exhibit. All items are rated on a 3-point scale: *not true, somewhat or sometimes true,* and *very true* or *often true.* The CBCL 1½–5 and C-TRF 1½–5 have identical subscales, with the exception of the Sleep Problems subscale, which is only on the CBCL 1½–5 (see Table 2.3). The individual subscales are summed to form broadband scales (Internalizing and Externalizing Problems) as well as a Total Problem score. A new feature on these measures is the use of DSM-oriented scales, which include items that were rated by psychologists and psychiatrists as being consistent with DSM-IV diagnostic categories. These DSM-oriented scales include Affective Problems, Anxiety Problems, Pervasive Developmental Problems, Attention-Deficit/Hyperactivity Problems, and Oppositional Defiant Problems. The CBCL 1½–5 also includes a Language Development Survey (LDS) to aid in the identification of language delays. A Spanish version of the CBCL 1½–5 rating form also is available. According to the manual, both of these scales have strong psychometric properties. However, because these versions of the scale are new, there is little outside research on their reliability and validity.

Behavior Assessment System for Children

The Behavior Assessment System for Children (BASC) is a comprehensive rating-scale system designed to assess problem behaviors in children and adolescents (Reynolds & Kamphaus, 1992). It includes both parent and teacher scales, with separate forms available to assess children in three age groups: 4–5, 6–11, and 12–18. The BASC scales for ages 6–11 and 12–18 were both well-normed and have good technical adequacy (Reynolds & Kamphaus, 1992). The Parent Rating Scale—Preschool version (PRS-P; normed on 309 children) and the Teacher Rating Scale—Preschool version (TRS-P; normed on 333 children) are highlighted here.

TABLE 2.3. CBCL and C-TRF 1½–5 Scales

Total Problems	DSM-Oriented Scales
Internalizing Problems	Affective Problems
Externalizing Problems	Anxiety Problems
	Pervasive Developmental Problems
Emotionally Reactive	Attention-Deficit/Hyperactivity Problems
Anxious/Depressed	Oppositional Defiant Problems
Somatic Complaints	
Withdrawn	
Attention Problems	
Aggressive Behavior	
Sleep Problems (CBCL only)	

The PRS-P contains 131 items, and the TRS-P contains 109 items. All items are rated as occurring *never, sometimes, often,* or *almost always.* Both scales have empirically derived composite scores and subscale scores that address a wide array of emotional and behavioral problems (see Table 2.4). Reliability and validity (including internal consistency reliability, short-term test–retest reliability, and convergent validity) are moderate to strong, as reported in the BASC manual. Fewer independent studies have been conducted with the BASC preschool version than with the older age-range versions of the scale. However, because of the overall strengths of the BASC system and the well-constructed composite and subscale scores, the TRS-P and the PRS-P appear to be very promising additions to the instrumentation available to assess this younger age group.

Conners' Rating Scales

The Conners' Rating Scales, and the new update, the Conners' Rating Scales—Revised (CRS-R; Conners, 1997), have been used for years to detect problem behaviors in children and adolescents. A unique feature of the Conners' system is that teacher, parent, and self-report scales are available in both long and short versions. For the parent and teacher forms, separate norms are available for boys and girls, in three-year age intervals, for children ages 3–17. The long versions of the Conners' scales—the Conners' Parent Rating Scale—Revised: Long Form (CPRS-R:L) and the Conners' Teacher Rating Scale—Revised: Long Form (CTRS-R:L)—each contains the same scales, with the exception of the Psychosomatic subscale that appears only on the parent version (see Table 2.5). The CPRS-R:L contains 80 items, and the CTRS-R:L contains 59 items. The Conners' Parent Rating Scale—Revised: Short Form (CPRS-R:S) and the Conners' Teacher Rating Scale—Revised: Short Form (CTRS-R:S) each contains four subscales that are approximately one-third to one-half the length of their longer counterparts: 27 items comprise the CPRS-R:S, and 28 comprise the CTRS-R:S. Parents and teachers are asked to consider the child's behaviors during the past month and rate their occurrence on a 4-point scale (*not at all true, just a little true, pretty much true,* or *very much true*).

Reliability and validity of the revised Conners' scales, as reported in the manual, are considered adequate to excellent. The standardization sample for the new CRS system is extremely large, with over 8,000 total normative cases. However, the normative groups for

---

TABLE 2.4. BASC PRS-P and TRS-P Scales

Externalizing Problems	Other Problems
Hyperactivity	Atypicality
Aggression	Withdrawal
	Attention Problems
Internalizing Problems	
Anxiety	Behavioral Symptoms Index
Depression	
Somatization	Adaptive Skills
	Adaptability
	Social Skills

TABLE 2.5. Conners' Rating Scales—Revised

CPRS-R:L and CTRS-R:L	CPRS-R:S and CTRS-R:S
Oppositional	Oppositional
Cognitive Problems/Inattention	Cognitive Problems/Inattention
Hyperactivity	Hyperactivity
Anxious–Shy	ADHD Index
Perfectionism	
Social Problems	
Psychosomatic (on parent version only)	
Conners' Global Index	
Restless–Impulsive	
Emotional Liability	
ADHD Index	
DSM-IV Symptoms Subscales	
DSM-IV Inattentive	
DSM-IV Hyperactive–Impulsive	

the 3–5-year-olds are considerably smaller than those for the older age ranges (109 for the CTRS-R:S; 198 for the CTRS-R:L; 303 for the CPRS-R:S; 375 for the CPRS-R:L). These scales can be used as general screeners for behavioral difficulties and can provide more focused assessment of children with attentional and hyperactive symptoms.

Preschool and Kindergarten Behavior Scales

The Preschool and Kindergarten Behavior Scales (PKBS; Merrell, 1994) is a 76-item behavior rating scale designed to measure social skills and social–emotional problem behaviors in children ages 3–6. This instrument can be completed by parents, teachers, daycare providers, or others who are familiar with the child's behavior.

The PKBS items were designed specifically to reflect the unique social and behavioral aspects of the preschool and kindergarten developmental period. The PKBS was developed with a national normative sample of over 2,800 children and has good psychometric properties, including adequate reliability and validity (Merrell, 1994). The items on the PKBS comprise two separate scales: a 34-item Social Skills Scale, and a 42-item Problem Behavior Scale. The subscales on the Social Skills Scale include Social Competence, Social Interaction, and Social Independence. The Problem Behavior Scale includes Self-Centered/Explosive, Anxiety/Somatic Problems, Antisocial/Aggressive, Attention Problems/Overactive, and Social Withdrawal. The PKBS is a useful tool for assessing general problem behaviors and social skills in young children, particularly those exhibiting the typical problems seen in daycares, preschools, and other classroom settings. For assessing children with severe problem behaviors of lower frequency, such as those exhibited by children in clinical settings, a scale such as the CBCL may be more appropriate.

Eyberg Child Behavior Inventory

The Eyberg Child Behavior Inventory (ECBI; Eyberg & Ross, 1978) is a 36-item parent rating scale used with children age 2 and older. The items reflect common behavior problems seen in children. Parents are asked to rate each item on a 7-point scale to indicate how often each behavior occurs. They also indicate with a "yes" or "no" rating whether each behavior is a problem for them. The ratings of behavior frequency are summed to create an Intensity Score, and the "yes" responses are summed to create a Problem Score. The ECBI is simple and quick to use (Kamphaus & Frick, 1996) and has been found to be particularly useful for identifying parents who have unusually high or low expectations for their child (Hembree-Kigin & McNeil, 1995). Although there is evidence that supports the ECBI's reliability and validity, there is also data which suggests the ECBI does not measure one single construct and may be best used as a measure of identifying treatment objectives and evaluating treatment outcome (Kamphaus & Frick, 1996).

A teacher version of this instrument (the Sutter–Eyberg Student Behavior Inventory; SESBI) also exists. The SESBI contains 36 items rated in the same manner as those on the ECBI, but these items have been reworded so that they are more appropriate for a school setting. Research conducted, to date, on this instrument supports its psychometric properties for use with preschool- and school-age children (Hembree-Kigin & McNeil, 1995; McMahon & Estes, 1997).

Social Skills Rating System

The Social Skills Rating System (SSRS; Gresham & Elliot, 1990) is a comprehensive social skills assessment system that includes parent and teacher preschool-age rating forms for use with children ages 3–5. The SSRS includes a variety of age ranges and assessment instruments; however, only the preschool forms are reviewed here. The parent and teacher preschool forms contain similar items that are rated on a 3-point scale to indicate how often each behavior occurs and how necessary the behavior is for social success. The forms also include a brief 10-item problem behavior screen to help determine if further assessment of behavioral problems is warranted. The parent form contains 39 social skills items, and the teacher form includes 30 items. Both versions include empirically derived subscales, including Cooperation, Assertion, and Self-Control in the social skills area, and Internalizing and Externalizing subscales in the problem behavior screening area.

The preschool forms of the SSRS were normed on 212 ratings for the teacher form and 193 ratings for the parent form. As reported in the manual, the psychometric properties for the overall SSRS are strong, though little evidence specifically related to the preschool forms is offered. Coefficient alpha reliabilities are low to moderate for the preschool versions. Although the SSRS is one of the only comprehensive systems for assessing social skills in preschool-age children, further research on the psychometric properties of the preschool versions should be conducted.

Attention Deficit Disorder Evaluation Scale

The Attention Deficit Disorder Evaluation Scale, Second Edition (ADDES, 2nd edition; McCarney, 1995a, 1995b) is a behavior rating scale designed to assess ADHD symptoms in the childhood and adolescent populations (ages 3–20). The ADDES has a home and a school version, both of which contain Inattentive and Hyperactive–Impulsive subscales.

The items from these two scales are summed to create a total score. Parents and teachers rate the child on a 5-point Likert-based scale, ranging from 0 ("Does Not Engage in the Behavior") to 5 ("Behavior Occurs One to Several Times per Hour"). The reliability and validity of both the home and school version are adequate, as reported in the manuals.

The Early Childhood Attention Deficit Disorders Evaluation Scale (ECADDES; McCarney, 1995c, 1995d) was designed specifically to assess ADHD symptoms in young children ages 2–6. The format of the scale resembles that of the older age version, in which parents and teachers rate the child on a 5-point Likert-based scale. The ECADDES also contains two subscales, Inattentive and Hyperactive–Impulsive, in addition to a Total Score. Overall there appears to be adequate technical support for the scale included in the manual, though there is a great deal of overlap between the two subscales, as evidenced by the factor analysis reported in the manual.

ADHD-Symptoms Rating Scale

The ADHD-Symptoms Rating Scale (ADHD-SRS; Holland, Gimpel, & Merrell, 2001) is designed specifically to assess behaviors symptomatic of ADHD in children and adolescents age 5–18. Two subscale scores (Hyperactive–Impulsive and Inattentive) as well as a Total score are obtained, and norms are available for both home and school raters. The ADHD-SRS was normed on a national sample of more than 2,800 individuals, and the technical properties of the scale are strong as reported in the manual. However, because the ADHD-SRS is a relatively new instrument, little outside research on it has been conducted, though the factor structure of the scale has been replicated using confirmatory factor analysis procedures (Collett, Crowley, Gimpel, & Greenson, 2000). Currently the scale can be used with children as young as 5 years of age; a preschool version of the scale is in progress.

For the preschool version, four of the 56 items that are specific to school-age children (e.g., "Fails to complete school work or homework") were removed in order to make the content more appropriate to the preschool population. Psychometric properties of the 52-item version have been evaluated with a sample of approximately 400 children ages 3–5. Internal consistency reliabilities were high, and the total score on the ADHD-SRS correlated highly with similar subscales on the BASC preschool version (Phillips, Greenson, Collett, & Gimpel, 2002). Although exploratory factor analyses were run, it was not clear whether a two-factor (Inattention and Hyperactivity–Impulsivity) or one-factor solution was best. Clearly more research is needed on this instrument. In addition, a larger, more representative normative sample is needed before norms and standard scores can be developed. However, this instrument does show promise for use with the preschool population.

ADHD Rating Scale–IV

The ADHD Rating Scale–IV (DuPaul, Power, Anastopoulos, & Reid, 1998) is an 18-item rating scale based on the DSM-IV criteria for ADHD. A single rating form, with separate norms for home and school raters, is used. The ADHD Rating Scale–IV contains both an

Inattention Scale and a Hyperactivity–Impulsivity Scale, which are summed to obtain a Total Score. The scale was normed on 2,000 ratings each of parents and teachers of children between the ages of 5 and 18. The authors of the ADHD Rating Scale–IV report adequate test–retest reliability and internal consistency reliability for all three scores as well as adequate convergent and construct validity (DuPaul et al., 1998). Although this scale has been used in a research context with preschool-age children, there is currently no normative or psychometric data for this age group.

Limitations of Rating Scales

Although rating scales offer numerous advantages over other forms of assessment, there are limitations associated with their use. Two major sources of error, discussed here as "error variance" and "response bias," can reduce the accuracy of ratings and must be considered when interpreting rating-scale results.

There are four possible sources of error variance in rating scales: *temporal variance*, which refers to the tendency of behavior ratings to be only moderately consistent over time; *setting variance*, which refers to the situational specificity of behavior; *source variance*, which refers to the objectivity (or lack thereof) of the rater; and *instrument variance*, which refers to the slight variations among rating scales purportedly measuring similar constructs (Merrell, 1999). "Response bias," or the way in which the informant responds to items also can introduce error into rating scale results. Four common response sets, or biases, are: *error of central tendency*, when the rater tends to use only those points in the middle of the scale, avoiding the high and low ends; *error from the halo effect*, when the rater rates an individual positively or negatively on all items, because the individual possesses a positive or negative trait unrelated to the behavior being rated; and *error of leniency or severity*, in which a rater is overly generous or overly severe and tends to rate all individuals mainly at the high or low ends of the scale (Anastasi, 1997). These types of response bias are present in varying degrees in all behavior rating scales.

Although the problems resulting from error variance are inherent in rating scales, there are ways to minimize their effects. Rating scales should never be used as the sole basis for making a diagnosis or placement/classification decision. Instead, rating scales should be part of a multimethod, multisource, multisetting assessment designed to obtain aggregated assessment information. By obtaining aggregated information, error variance should be minimized (Merrell, 1999).

DIRECT OBSERVATION

Observation is one of the most valuable tools in the assessment of young children. Because young children communicate more through behavior than words, observation serves as a cornerstone of psychological assessment when evaluating the social, emotional, and behavioral functioning of this age group. Prior to observing a child, it is important to define the behaviors to be observed and to consider whether to use informal or formal observational methods.

Defining Observable Behaviors

In order to observe behavior in a manner that leads to useful information, the "target behavior," or the behavior to be evaluated, must be clearly identified. Broad constructs, such as "aggressive," "hyperactive," "poor social skills," "anxious," "friendly," etc., must be defined, so that the observer and the teacher, daycare worker, or parent have a common understanding of what specific behaviors to observe. In other words, vague psychological terms must be broken down into measurable components so that they are "operationally defined" (Kazdin, 2001). For example, if a child is described by his/her preschool teacher as being "hyper" in the classroom, the observer must interview the teacher more thoroughly to understand specifically what behaviors mean "hyper" to that teacher. Once the observer gathers specific descriptors of that behavior from the teacher (e.g., "out of seat during seat time," "climbing on chairs," "fidgeting in seat," "throwing classroom materials"), then he/she can track those behaviors more precisely and accurately during the observation.

Structured Observations

Structured observations, including formal and informal coding systems, can be helpful in identifying and tracking problem behaviors in the school, home, or daycare setting. Before any observation is conducted, the observer should have already interviewed the teacher, daycare provider, and/or parent to obtain more information on the child's referral problem. In addition, the behaviors to be observed should be operationally defined.

The behaviors of young children are often variable across settings, times, and individuals. Ideally, the observer would watch the child at different times of the day and while the child is engaged in different activities. The observer should attempt to see the child as many times as necessary to observe a representative range of behaviors and affective states. In addition, the child should be observed interacting with different peers and/or adults across multiple settings, in order to obtain the most complete picture of his/her behaviors (Benham, 2000).

Naturalistic observations—observing the child in his/her natural environment, such as the school or daycare—offer advantages over other observational methods. In naturalistic observations the child is able to engage in normal daily activities in which his/her targeted behaviors naturally occur. Naturalistic observations also provide the observer with the opportunity to determine *antecedents* (what happens right before the behavior occurs) and *consequences* (what happens right after the behavior occurs) that may be maintaining the child's behaviors (see "Functional Analysis" later in this chapter). During this type of observation, it is important that the observer remain as unobtrusive as possible, so that the child is not influenced by his/her presence (Merrell, 1999).

In addition to observing the child's behavior, it is important to attend to setting variables that may be related to the behaviors of concern. Important elements of the setting to pay attention to include: (1) the adult's interactions with the children; (2) possible distractions or outside noises; (3) what happens prior to and after the child exhibits the problem behavior; and (4) the physical setting the child is in, including the amount of space available to the child, the child's proximity to other children throughout the day, and the materials available in the setting.

After completing the observation, the observer should talk with the teacher/daycare worker about his/her perceptions of the child's behaviors during the observation period. In particular, the observer should ask the teacher/daycare worker if the behaviors exhibited by the child during the observation are representative of his/her usual behaviors in that setting. The observer also should note whether the teacher/daycare provider seems to be especially lenient or critical of the child and if his/her observations match the observer's.

Informal, Structured Observation Methods

For the purposes of this book, *informal observation* means that a formal, published observational system was not used, though coding charts or other aids may have been used. As mentioned above, the first step in conducting an observation is to operationally define the behaviors that will be observed. Once this is done, the observer must choose how to record the data. A variety of recording methods have been identified and summarized (Kazdin, 2001; Merrell, 1999). Here we review those most likely to be used when observing young children. A summary of these selected techniques is provided in Table 2.6. To illustrate each of these techniques, the example of a child screaming in class (e.g., raising his/her voice above peers and/or what is expected in that particular classroom setting) is used.

Using the *event or frequency recording* procedure, the observer would record the number of times a specific behavior occurs over the length of the observation—in our example, the number of times the child screams in class during a 20-minute observation session. The advantages of this system are that it is easy to use (the observer makes

TABLE 2.6. Observation Coding Procedures

Technique	Definition	Example
Event/frequency recording	Record the number of times the specific behavior occurs over length of the observation	Record number of times child screams
Duration recording	Record the length of time a behavior occurs	Record length of time child screams
Interval recording		
Partial-interval recording	Record the behavior if it occurred at any point during the interval	Record screaming if child screams at any time during the interval
Whole-interval recording	Record the behavior only if it occurred during the entire interval	Record screaming only if the child screams throughout the entire interval
Momentary time sampling	Record the behavior at exact intervals in time	Look at child every 15 seconds; if child is screaming at that instant, record as screaming

checkmarks or uses a simple counter to track when the behavior occurs), and it can be used to determine antecedents and consequences of the child's behavior (see upcoming section on functional analysis). A disadvantage of this method is that it cannot easily be used with behaviors that do not have a clear beginning and end (e.g., fidgeting could be difficult to record with this technique, as it often does not have a clear beginning or end).

When using *duration recording,* the observer would record the length of time a behavior occurs. Both total duration (total time the child screamed during the observation period; e.g., 6 of the 20 minutes) and duration per event (the length of time the child screamed each time it occurred; e.g., one scream that was 1 minute, and another that was 5 minutes) can be calculated. The duration recording procedure has the advantage of being simple to conduct using a wall clock or stopwatch, though it is not helpful for behaviors without a clear beginning or end (e.g., fidgeting in seat) and may be less useful for behaviors that are short in duration.

If an observer were using *interval recording,* he/she would record the presence or absence of a given response within a certain time interval. In our example, the 20-minute observational period would be divided into short intervals of, perhaps, 30 seconds each, and the behavior would be recorded if the child screams (1) at any time during the interval (*partial-interval recording*) or (2) during the entire interval (*whole-interval recording*). Interval recording techniques are a good choice for behaviors that are not clearly discrete or for behaviors that occur at a moderate but steady rate (e.g., thumb sucking). A disadvantage of the techniques is that they require the observer's complete attention on the child. Therefore, these techniques are more difficult to use reliably and would be particularly difficult for a teacher or other staff member to do if he/she also had to attend to other matters in the classroom. An example of an interval recording form is included in Figure 2.3.

The *momentary time sampling* procedure is a type of interval recording, but it does not require the observer to monitor the whole interval. Using this procedure, the observer divides the observation session into equal intervals, as with the interval recording methods. However, the behavior would be counted as occurring only if it is emitted at the moment the interval terminates. For example, with a 15-second interval, the behavior would be recorded as occurring or not occurring once every 15 seconds. In our example, the child would be recorded as screaming in class only if the behavior was occurring at the moment the interval (e.g., 15-second period) ended. This technique requires only one observation per interval, and it is useful for behaviors that are apt to persist. However, some important, lower frequency behaviors may be missed when using this procedure.

Once the observer has completed his/her observations of the child, it is important to determine the significance of the data. Obviously, if the child's behaviors are dangerous or significantly disruptive, they would be considered problematic and would require some form of immediate intervention. However, because other behaviors, such as difficulty staying seated or fidgeting, are common among preschoolers and kindergartners, it would be important to determine if these behaviors are atypical in comparison to peers or problematic given the requirements of the setting in which the child was observed. To help determine if a child's behaviors are more severe than his/her peers, the observer should also record the same behaviors of several randomly selected peers from the child's class, daycare, or other setting.

BEHAVIOR RECORDING FORM

Child's name: Jane Smith **Date:** August 7th
Observer: Joe Jones **Location observed:** Kindergarten
Activity observed: Story Time & Rug Time **Start/stop time:** 9:30–9:45 A.M.
Interval length/type: 30 seconds/partial interval recording

Interval	Screaming	Out of area	Hitting others
1	X		
2		X	X
3		X	
4	X		
5	X		
6			
7			
8			
9		X	
10		X	
11			
12			
13			
14			
15	X		X
16			
17			
18			
19			
20		X	
21		X	
22	X	X	
23			
24			
25			
26	X		
27	X		
28			
29			
30		X	

FIGURE 2.3. Example of the interval recording procedure.

Informal Observations by Parents or Teachers

Often a clinician will ask parents or teachers to keep track of behavior problems they are seeing in the home/classroom. These observations may have some structure to them (e.g., a recording form is often used) but are often less structured than those the clinician would do him/herself. These observations can be particularly helpful in the home setting. Rarely does a clinician go into the home to observe behaviors. Having a parent track behaviors in the home can provide valuable information regarding how often the behaviors of concern are occurring in this setting. When asking parents or teachers to track behaviors, a simple frequency count method is typically used. Figure 2.4 shows an example of a "behavior log" that could be used by parents to track the occurrence of some of the more common disruptive behaviors seen in the home environment.

Functional Assessment

A functional assessment of behavior involves determining the "purpose" of the behavior in terms of what is reinforcing and maintaining it. As part of a functional assessment, an A-B-C structure to observe behavior is used: *A* is the antecedent of the behavior, *B* is the behavior, and *C* is the consequence of the behavior. In general, functional assessments should identify (1) the antecedent conditions that give rise to the problem behavior; (2) the source of reinforcement that should be eliminated; (3) the general reinforcement contingency that will form the basis for treatment of the behavior problem; and (4) the monitoring of progress and follow-up to ensure the treatment was successful (Hawkins, 1979). By determining the function of a behavior and matching interventions to this function, the effectiveness of treatments should be increased.

Researchers have noted that problem behaviors generally serve one of several functions: children receive social attention (from peers or teachers); children are able to escape or avoid a task; sensory reinforcement is provided; or access to a tangible reinforcer is obtained (Gresham & Lambros, 1998). Knowing the function of the behavior can help prevent the problem behavior from being inadvertently reinforced. For example, if a functional assessment determines that a child misbehaves to escape participation in story time, sending the child to time-out for misbehaving in this situation would not be appropriate and would likely reinforce the misbehavior, because it allows the child to escape the story time. Instead, inappropriate behaviors can be ignored and the child can be positively reinforced for engaging in story time.

Although observational methods are often used to obtain the information needed for a functional assessment, interviews with parents and teachers also help identify the antecedents and consequences of the behavior (e.g., ask the parent what he/she does after the child misbehaves), as can asking parents/teachers to use a behavior log (such as the one in Figure 2.5) to record what happens before and after the problem behavior occurs. When conducting an observation to identify the possible function of a targeted behavior, the observer would document the antecedents of the misbehavior (e.g., screaming), or what happens right before the child begins to scream (e.g., the child is engaged in a solitary activity), as well as the consequences of the child's screaming (e.g., the child gets attention from the teacher and the screaming stops). In this example (assuming this pattern is consistent across time), it appears that the child's behavior is being maintained by attention, so the intervention should focus on decreasing attention for screaming and increasing attention for appropriate talking.

BEHAVIOR LOG

Child's Name _____

Behaviors should be recorded for at least 3 days during the time between dinnertime and bedtime.

If no problem behaviors occurred on a certain day, make sure to indicate so by writing either a "0" or "no behaviors" in the appropriate column.

In Hours column please record the number of hours for which you recorded behaviors.

Date	Hours	Noncompliance	Physical Aggression	Temper Tantrums
Example: 1-1-02	Example: 3	Example: III	Example: 0	Example: IIII

FIGURE 2.4. Home behavior log. From Gretchen A. Gimpel and Melissa L. Holland (2003). Copyright by The Guilford Press. Permission to photocopy this figure is granted to purchasers of this book for personal use only (see copyright page for details).

BEHAVIOR LOG

Behavior: _____   Child: _____

Date	Time	Description of behavior	Situation in which behavior occurred	What happened after behavior occurred

FIGURE 2.5. Functional analysis behavior log. From Gretchen A. Gimpel and Melissa L. Holland (2003). Copyright by The Guilford Press. Permission to photocopy this figure is granted to purchasers of this book for personal use only (see copyright page for details).

Formal Observations

Though there are numerous formal observational systems designed to provide information on children's behaviors in naturalistic settings (e.g., home, school, or daycare), few focus specifically on the young child. One measure that does include observations of preschool and kindergarten children is the Early Screening Project (ESP; Walker, Severson, & Feil, 1995). The ESP includes observations of young children's behaviors through its Social Behavior Observations component. The ESP observations are designed to provide information on children's social behaviors and, in particular, children's social interactions with peers and adults. A duration recording technique is used to record the amount of time the observed child is engaged in *prosocial behaviors,* such as playing well with others; *negative social behaviors,* such as verbal misbehaviors, disobeying rules, or throwing tantrums; or *nonsocial behavior,* such as solitary play. Normative data are available, enabling the observer to compare the child being observed with other children his/her age to determine if the problem behaviors are significant.

CHAPTER SUMMARY

The social and emotional assessment of young children is still a relatively new domain. Measures and techniques specifically for use with preschool- and kindergarten-age children are less prevalent and often less psychometrically sophisticated than those available for use with older children. Advancements during the recent years have included behavior rating scales designed specifically to assess the problem behaviors of young children, and research on observational methods and interviewing techniques for use with the preschool- and kindergarten-age child. In general, the best practice for assessing the young child involves integrating information from various sources and measures in order to gain the most complete and accurate diagnostic picture of the child without stigmatizing or overpathologizing normal childhood behaviors.

3

Treatment of Externalizing/
Acting-Out Problems

As noted in Chapter 1, the three DSM-IV disorders that comprise the externalizing problems include conduct disorder (CD), oppositional defiant disorder (ODD), and attention-deficit/hyperactivity disorder (ADHD). However, many preschool- and kindergarten-age children with disruptive behaviors do not receive a formal DSM diagnosis. These children are often referred by parents or teachers who are having difficulties managing behaviors such as noncompliance, temper tantrums, aggression, and whining. As stated in Chapter 1, for some children these behaviors are a normal and temporary part of childhood. For other children, though, these behaviors are indicative of long-term problems. Although it can be difficult to predict which children will continue to have problems and which will not, several of the predictors of problem behavior stability are related to parenting or family factors. For example, parenting behaviors that involve warmth and clear limit setting are more likely to lead to prosocial behaviors in children, whereas negative or uninvolved parenting behaviors are more likely to lead to behavioral difficulties in children (Campbell, 1997). Given these findings, one of the most common interventions for externalizing child behavior problems is parent training, which focuses on increasing parental responsiveness and consistency.

Numerous studies support the use of parent training as an intervention for general conduct problems in children of varying ages (Serketich & Dumas, 1996). A growing body of research also supports the use of both individual (e.g., Schuhman, Foote, Eyberg, Boggs, & Algina, 1998) and group (e.g., Webster-Stratton & Hammond, 1997) parent training for families of preschool-age children who have disruptive behavior disorders. Studies also have supported the use of parent training for preschool children with ADHD, in both group (Pisterman et al., 1989) and individual (Sonuga-Barke, Daley, Thompson, Laver-Bradbury, & Weeks, 2001) settings. In addition to improving parenting skills and reducing child disruptive behaviors, parent training programs may lead to other positive changes in parent and family functioning (e.g., reduced parental depression, improved family relations) (Kazdin & Wassell, 2000), although research on such effects is less consistent.

Although parent training is the most researched intervention for disruptive behaviors, school-based behavioral interventions and child-focused social skills interventions also have received some empirical support. This chapter begins with a comprehensive overview of parent training methods, followed by a review of school-based and social skills interventions. The chapter ends with a discussion of comprehensive early intervention/prevention programs that have been developed in an attempt to ameliorate the long-term negative effects of conduct problems.

PARENT TRAINING AS AN INTERVENTION FOR EXTERNALIZING PROBLEMS

Overview

Behaviorally oriented parent training programs are based on operant conditioning procedures and social learning theory. Operant conditioning procedures involve the application of consequences following a behavior, in order to increase or decrease the likelihood of that behavior recurring. For example, a child who offers to share his/her toys is praised; a child who grabs toys from a playmate is sent to time-out. These programs assume that the child's behavior is related to interactions the child has with significant others (e.g., parents) and that to change the child's behaviors, one must first change the behavior of those significant others. Thus, in parent training, the clinician works directly with parents to help them acquire skills that better address the problem behaviors exhibited by their child. Although the child is often present in parent training sessions, the clinician does not work individually with the child.

The current behavioral parent training programs are based on a model, originally developed by Hanf (1969), which involves a two-part program. In the first part of the program, parents are taught to use positive skills to increase appropriate child behaviors. These skills are typically taught in a play-based context and involve teaching parents to administer positive attention and praise. After mastering the positive skills, parents are taught to give effective commands to their children and to use effective methods of discipline (typically, time-out). Most behavioral parent training programs today continue to use this model, including the presentation of the positive component prior to introducing the discipline component. However, there is little research on the effects of ordering, and at least one study has indicated order does not influence treatment outcome (Eisenstadt, Eyberg, McNeil, Newcomb, & Funderburk, 1993). However, it is important that parents learn that it is ineffective to use discipline skills in isolation and that they also need to provide positive responses for appropriate behaviors.

Active training methods are used to teach parenting skills. Skills are first taught didactically, through verbal explanations to parents. In addition, handouts that describe the skills and their application are provided, and the skills are then modeled in session by the clinician. Ideally this is done with the referred child present, although videotaped models also may be used. For example, parents may be shown a videotape of one parent using the skills appropriately and another using the skills inappropriately, so that they can observe the difference in the application of the skills as well as the response of the child. Following the initial modeling, parents practice the skills in session and receive feedback from the clinician. Parents are also assigned homework that involves practicing the new skills in the home environment and monitoring their progress. The feedback or coaching aspect of parent training is important in helping parents learn how to use the skills effectively. When initially learning a skill, parents may apply it inappropriately, or they may have difficulties with the application of the skill that were not anticipated prior to practice. This observation and coaching can help address these problems as they arise. In addition, directly observing the parent using the skills assists the clinician in obtaining an accurate picture of the parent's skill level. When providing feedback, it is important that the clinician provide positive responses on what parents are doing well, in addition to corrective feedback.

Initial Considerations

Although parent training is often an effective intervention for families who have a child displaying disruptive and noncompliant behaviors, it is not appropriate for all families. Before deciding to use parent training, several factors must be considered. Often an initial consideration is the age of the child. Parent training programs can be used with parents of children of varying ages, although most are focused on parents of children rather than adolescents. The preschool age range is typically considered the ideal time to intervene, and many parent training programs are geared specifically toward the parenting of preschool and early elementary school-age children (e.g., Hembree-Kigin & McNeil, 1995). Parent training programs are typically not used with parents of very young children (under the age of 2), although with significant modifications it would be possible to accommodate parents of this age group.

Parent-related factors such as socioeconomic status, parental psychopathology, marital problems, and level of social support have all been found to influence the effectiveness of parent training programs (Kazdin, 1993, 1997). Thus it is important to ask about such factors as part of a comprehensive intake assessment. Providing additional services in order to more completely address their needs may be appropriate for some families. For example, if a parent is experiencing depression, or a couple is having marital problems, it would be appropriate to refer these families for additional services. Children also may require additional services, such as programs targeting school behavior or medications. Comprehensive services targeting both parent and child issues may address the needs of the family more completely and thereby increase the overall effectiveness of parent training (Dadds, Schwartz, & Sanders, 1987; Webster-Stratton, 1994).

Parental motivation also plays a key role in the outcome of parent training programs and should be assessed prior to beginning the training. Some parents react negatively to parent training because of the focus on working with the parents rather than with the child. When parents initially seek services, they often expect the clinician to meet with their child individually, and they do not expect to be extensively involved in the intervention. Some parents may perceive parent training (with its focus on the parents) as an insult to their parenting skills. Other parents may simply not have the time or energy to devote to parent training. Often, providing parents with a rationale for the use of parent training can resolve some of these issues and help prevent confusion about services (which will hopefully reduce dropout rates).

When providing a rationale for parent training, it is important to emphasize that such training can be very effective in managing children who exhibit conduct problems, and that early intervention is central to preventing the problems from worsening over time. It is important to link the parents' behavior with the child's behavior without blaming the parents for the child's inappropriate reactions. Explaining to parents that their behaviors can influence their child's behaviors, and that by changing their behaviors, they can improve their child's behaviors is often effective. Children with conduct problems usually have different behavior patterns from those of other children, and thus parents need to learn different ways to interact with them to help decrease the negative behaviors and increase the positive ones. In addition, it should be acknowledged that parenting, in general, can be stressful, and that parenting a child with conduct problems is even more stressful. Because of this added stress, parents may react with frustration in ways that only increase negative child behaviors. Changing parenting behaviors in order to change child behaviors should lead to less stressful and more positive parent–child interactions.

Conducting Parent Training

In the following sections, a typical behavioral parent training program is outlined. This program is very similar to parent training programs discussed by others (e.g., Barkley, 1997; Hembree-Kigin & McNeil, 1995; Schroeder & Gordan, 2002): like most behavioral parent training programs, it is based on the two-part model of teaching positive responses and discipline skills. An outline of the steps involved in the program is provided in Table 3.1.

TABLE 3.1. Outline of Behavioral Parent Training Treatment Components

Providing explanation and overview of behavioral terminology
Giving positive attention for appropriate behaviors
Giving effective commands
Using discipline techniques for inappropriate behaviors
    Time-out
    Use of privileges
Managing behaviors in public places (generalization of skills)
Maintenance phase (e.g., booster sessions)

Explaining Behavioral Principles

Because behavioral parent training is based on operant conditioning principles, it is important for parents to understand these principles. If parents do not understand why they are implementing a skill in a certain way, it is less likely that they will continue to implement the skill after the termination of therapy services, and it is less likely that they will be able to problem solve as they encounter new behavior problems. Obviously, too much theoretical detail may be overwhelming for parents, but a brief explanation of key behavioral principles can be quite helpful. Parents are given a handout (see Figure 3.1) that contains succinct explanations of behavioral principles such as positive and negative reinforcement, response cost, and extinction. The clinician should go over this handout with the parents and attempt to elicit examples of the child's behavior to help illustrate these principles. It is often helpful for the clinician to provide an example and then ask the parent for an additional example, using an interaction the parent has recently had with the child.

Positive Reinforcement for Appropriate Behaviors

In the positive reinforcement phase of parent training, parents are taught to attend to and praise appropriate behaviors exhibited by their child. Parents of children with behavior problems are usually so overwhelmed by the need to monitor (and attempt to decrease) their children's negative behaviors that they neglect to notice the appropriate behaviors. This type of one-sided interaction can lead to the coercive parenting cycle described in Chapter 1. By attending to appropriate behaviors, parents (1) increase the likelihood that these behaviors will increase in frequency and (2) they help teach the child which behaviors he/she *should* do rather than focusing solely on what the child should *not* do. This positive part of parent training can help set the stage for a more positive and enjoyable parent–child relationship overall. In addition, positive feedback may help increase the child's self-esteem, which is a common concern for parents.

These positive attending skills are taught and practiced in the context of child-focused play situations that are often referred to as the "Child's Game" or "Time-In." Two to four different types of age-appropriate toys that promote constructive, interactive play should be available for this activity. Legos, wooden blocks, Tinker Toys, Lincoln Logs, and drawing materials are commonly used. Toys that should be avoided are those that do not allow for spontaneous interactions between the child and parent, and those that have the potential to promote aggressive play. For example, board games should be avoided because of the structured rules involved. During this positive playtime, the parent's attention should be focused completely on the child, and the child should be allowed to lead the play. In order to keep the play child-focused, parents are told to refrain from asking questions, giving commands, or being critical. They also are instructed to ignore instances of minor misbehavior. (For major misbehaviors, parents are instructed to end playtime.) During this playtime, parents are told to (1) describe what the child is doing (e.g., "You're putting the yellow block on top of the blue block."), (2) reflect verbal statements the child makes (e.g., after the child says, "I like blue," the parent might say, "You like blue. I do too. Blue is a pretty color."), and (3) praise the child for appropriate behaviors. Parents should be

BEHAVIORAL TERMINOLOGY AND GUIDELINES

Children (and adults) often act according to certain behavioral principles. Understanding these principles and the ways they work can help you understand why your child behaves the way he/she does. Applying skills based on these principles will help you increase your child's good behaviors and decrease his/her negative behaviors. Many of these principles will sound like common sense, while others may not. Just remember that all of them have been studied extensively and have been shown to be effective.

ABCs of Behavior

A = antecedent—what is happening <u>before</u> a behavior occurs

B = behavior—the actual behavior that occurs

C = consequence—what happens <u>after</u> the behavior occurs. If the consequence is good, the behavior is more likely to happen again; if the consequence is bad the behavior is less likely to happen again.

Let's look at the ABCs using an example. A child is in a store with his mother and sees the candy rack at the checkout counter and begins pestering his mother for candy. The antecedent, or "A," would be seeing candy in the checkout aisle. The behavior, or "B," would be asking or pestering for candy. If the consequence, or "C," is that the mother buys the child candy, the child will be more likely to behave this way in the future in the same situation. But, if the consequence is that the mother does not buy the child candy and ignores the pestering, the child will be less likely to try this again in the future.

Reinforcement

Positive Reinforcement. This type of reinforcement involves giving a pleasant consequence to increase a behavior. Consequences that increase behaviors are called **reinforcers**. Reinforcers differ from child to child. To determine reinforcers for your child, think about what your child likes. Reinforcers include toys and money as well as attention and praise. Some unpleasant things can also be reinforcers. For example, children are often reinforced by parental attention, and even negative parental attention (yelling) may increase behaviors.

For reinforcers (and all consequences) to be most effective, they must occur **immediately** after a behavior.

Negative Reinforcement. This is also called **escape**. Escape involves taking away something unpleasant to increase a behavior. For example, a child who does not like math class may act out in math class and get sent to the principal's office. In this case, being sent to the principal's office is reinforcing to the child because he/she gets to escape from math (an unpleasant activity). This child is then more likely to act out in math class in the future.

Often parents and children get in a pattern of negative reinforcement. For example, your child may whine to get out cleaning his/her room (escape a negative task). Because whining is unpleasant to you, you give in and allow your child not to clean his/her room. The next time your child whines,

(continued)

FIGURE 3.1. Behavioral terminology and guidelines. From Gretchen A. Gimpel and Melissa L. Holland (2003). Copyright by The Guilford Press. Permission to photocopy this figure is granted to purchasers of this book for personal use only (see copyright page for details).

you will be more likely to do the same thing because you have been negatively reinforced (the unpleasant whining stops) for giving in. In addition, your child has been negatively reinforced by your withdrawal of the negative task. Thus your child is more likely to whine again in the future.

Extinction

Extinction can be used to decrease behaviors. This involves **not** reinforcing a behavior that was previously reinforced. For example, if your child cries and complains about going to school in the morning, and you had been allowing him/her to stay home but now start ignoring the crying and complaining and make your child go to school, eventually he/she will stop complaining because this behavior is no longer reinforced.

Extinction Burst

When using extinction, the behavior often gets worse before it gets better. This is called an **extinction burst**. If you begin ignoring your child's complaining, you can expect longer, louder complaining at first. However, if you continue to ignore the complaining, it will stop. It is very important that you continue with the ignoring, even as the complaining worsens. If you initially ignore the complaining but give in when it becomes too bothersome, you will have taught your child that if he/she complains long enough, he/she will get his/her way. In reality, you will have made matters worse! This is why you must be committed to using extinction before you begin.

Differential Reinforcement

When children misbehave, we can often change their behavior by reinforcing them for something we approve of and ignoring the misbehavior. This is called **differentially reinforcing other behavior**. For example, when your child is throwing toys (in an effort to get your attention), ignore the throwing behavior and once he/she does **any other** appropriate behavior, reinforce him/her for it quickly. For example, if he/she picks up a truck and rolls it on the floor, reinforce him/her for this appropriate activity. Keep reinforcing good behaviors and ignoring the inappropriate behaviors. This pattern of attending will stop the throwing and increase the behaviors you reinforce.

Punishment

Punishment also can be used decrease behaviors. Just like reinforcement, there are two types of punishment.

Type 1. This is when something unpleasant happens right after a behavior and reduces the chance the behavior will happen again. For example, a child who refuses to eat his vegetables is yelled at, and the next time he is presented with vegetables, he eats them.

Type 2 (Response Cost). This is removal of a positive reinforcer after a behavior occurs. For example, a teenager comes home late and has car privileges taken away. Because something is being taken away, the misbehavior "costs" the child something that is reinforcing to him/her.

Type 1 punishment may work immediately when you want a child to stop a behavior, but there are drawbacks to this method. Often when the punisher/punishment is absent, the behavior still occurs. Type 1 punishment also may make the punisher a feared person. In addition, using physical punishment in the home creates an environment for aggression and increases the chances that children will react in aggressive ways. Thus we do not recommended Type 1 punishment.

encouraged to use a combination of specific, labeled praise statements (e.g., "Thank you for handing me the block I needed. You shared very nicely without me even asking.") as well as general, unlabeled praise ("Great job!"). Because labeled praise statements are helpful in letting the child know specifically what it is the parent likes, it is important that parents incorporate such praise statements in their interactions with their child.

When teaching parents to use these positive, child-directed skills, the clinician explains the activity to the parents and provides a rationale for its use. Parents are also given a handout (see Figure 3.2) that contains a detailed description of this step. Once this activity has been explained to parents, the clinician should model the skills with the referred child, so that the parents can see how the skills are implemented. Although this activity sounds relatively easy to do, it is actually quite difficult in practice. Thus clinicians should make sure their skills are adequate before teaching and modeling these skills for the parents. In addition, it is important to acknowledge that parents often feel silly doing this at first (especially in the presence of the clinician) and that many parents have particular difficulties avoiding questions when first learning this "game." Because asking questions is a common way for adults to interact with children, parents often ask why they need to avoid questions during this positive time. The clinician should explain that the purpose of this play activity is for parents to overlearn positive attending skills and that anything that takes away from the child-directed nature of the activity should be avoided. Because questions tend to lead play and conversation, they are to be avoided during this time. However, parents should be assured that there is nothing wrong with asking questions of their child in their everyday interactions.

Once the skills have been modeled by the clinician, the parent should be encouraged to gradually join in the play. Eventually the clinician should allow the parent to take over the play with the child, and the clinician should coach the parent on his/her use of the child-directed skills. For example, if the parent asks a question (e.g., "These are colorful blocks, aren't they?") but does not realize the error, the clinician would point it out to the parent (e.g., "Oops, that was a question. Try just saying, 'Those are colorful blocks you're playing with.'") If the parent is having difficulties knowing what to say (i.e., there are long periods of silence), the clinician should encourage the parent to provide a description or praise statement (e.g., "Now would be a good time to tell Ella you like how she's sharing her crayons with you."). As mentioned above, it is important that the clinician also gives the parent positive feedback when the parent uses a skill well (e.g., "Nice job praising Sammy for sharing with you.").

In addition to coaching the parent on what he/she is saying, it is important to attend to and coach the parent on the way the statements are delivered. When first engaging in this activity, parents often sound unenthusiastic and have little inflection in their voices. It is extremely important that clinicians model enthusiasm when they are interacting with the child, and that they coach parents to be more enthusiastic if needed. Parents who are unenthusiastic or do not appear genuine will often have problems keeping their children engaged and interested in this activity, because children will pick up on their parents' lack of interest.

As homework, parents are instructed to practice these skills for at least 5 minutes per day and to track their practice as well as note any problems they encountered (see

PAYING POSITIVE ATTENTION TO YOUR CHILD'S GOOD BEHAVIOR

In order to increase your child's good behaviors, it is important to reinforce these behaviors by paying attention to them. In order to learn to attend to positive behavior, it is necessary to practice these skills. The best way to do this is in a play setting. Below are guidelines for conducting these play sessions. Although this program sounds easy to do, it if often difficult for parents at first. Don't be discouraged—just keep trying your best. Pretty soon, you'll see results!

1. **Select a time.** Select a 5–15-minute time period each day to play with your child. It is good to be consistent with the amount of time you spend with your child, so if you don't have much time, choose to play for only 5 minutes each night.

2. **Interact with just one child.** During this playtime, you should play with only one child at a time. You can engage in this activity with all of your children, but make sure to play with each child separately so that each child can enjoy one-on-one time with you. Choose a time for this activity when you will not be interrupted by your other children or when your spouse or a friend can entertain them.

3. **Select appropriate toys.** Select three or four different toys your child can play with during this special playtime. These toys should be constructive and nonviolent in nature (e.g., blocks, Legos, Lincoln Logs). Tell the child, "It's time for our special time," and allow the child to begin playing with the preselected toys.

4. **Use child-directed statements.** As you begin playing with your child, use the following types of verbalizations and interactions:

    a. **Descriptions.** Describe what your child is doing. This should be done in a genuine and enthusiastic manner and should focus on something specific the child is doing. Descriptions are used to indicate to your child that you find him/her and his/her play interesting.

    Examples of description statements include:

    "You put the blue block on top of the red block."
    "You've got a green crayon, and you're drawing a circle."
    "It looks like you're building a house with those Legos—you've got windows and a door."

    b. **Reflections.** When your child says something, reflect back what he/she said. This is another method of demonstrating to your child that you heard what he/she said and are interested in what was said. Reflections should not be direct "parroting" of what your child said but should convey the basic message to your child that you are listening.

    Examples of reflections include:

    Your child says: "I'm gonna draw a monster."
    You say: "You're going to draw a monster—I can't wait to see it."

(continued)

FIGURE 3.2. Paying positive attention to your child's good behavior. From Gretchen A. Gimpel and Melissa L. Holland (2003). Copyright by The Guilford Press. Permission to photocopy this figure is granted to purchasers of this book for personal use only (see copyright page for details).

Your child says: "Green is my favorite color."
You say: "You like green. That is a nice color."

c. **Praise/approval:** Provide your child with verbal praise for appropriate behaviors or positive feedback on what the child is doing. These statements should be genuine and at least half should be specific statements that indicate to your child the specific behavior of which you approve.

Examples of praise statements include:
"I like how still you're sitting in your chair."
"What a great drawing—you drew a really scary looking monster."

d. **Joining in/imitation.** Join in with what your child is doing. For example, if he/she is building towers with blocks, you should also build something with the blocks.

5. **Avoid directive statements.** Because this playtime is intended to be child-focused, you should avoid making any directive or critical statements that would take away from that focus. During your playtime, you should reframe from the following:

a. **Asking questions:** For example, "What are your drawing?"
b. **Giving commands:** For example, "Why don't you draw a picture of our house."
c. **Being critical:** For example, "That's not a very good picture of our house—our house is white, not red."

Questions, in particular, may be hard to eliminate—we are accustomed to interacting with children by asking questions. Although it is appropriate at many times to ask questions, in this context they would lead the play or conversation in the direction *you* want to go and require the child to respond to *you.* Thus, for this playtime to be completely child-directed and focused, reframe from asking questions.

6. Occasionally during this playtime, your child will misbehave. If this misbehavior is minor, simply turn away from the child. You can continue playing on your own (and describing what you are doing), but do not look at the child or make comments to the child until he/she begins to behave appropriately again. Once this occurs, immediately attend to your child. If the misbehavior continues or if the original misbehavior was severe, simply tell your child playtime is over.

Figure 3.3). If there are multiple children in the household, the parents should practice with only one child at a time. Parents are encouraged to use these skills with children other than the referred child, but each child should have his/her own time. If there are two parents in the household, it is ideal to have each parent practice these skills—again, though, they should do this independently.

These skills are practiced in session until parents have mastered their use. Some parent training programs have specific guidelines for determining when mastery of these techniques is achieved. For example, in Parent–Child Interaction Therapy (one of the specific behavioral parent training programs available), parents are considered to have mastered these skills when they can provide 25 descriptive and/or reflective statements, 15 praise statements, and no questions, commands, or criticisms within a 5-minute period (Hembree-Kigin & McNeil, 1995).

Giving Effective Commands and Using Appropriate Discipline Techniques

After mastering the positive attention component, parents are taught to give effective commands. It is important that parents learn how to give appropriate commands prior to the implementation of discipline strategies. Parents often give commands that make it difficult or impossible for the child to comply (e.g., providing a long string of different commands without giving the child time to comply in between commands; giving vague commands that do not give the child enough information about what he/she is expected to do). In addition, parents often phrase statements as commands but do not intend to follow through with a consequence if the child does not comply. Parents should be instructed to only give commands when they plan to follow through with an appropriate consequence for compliance or noncompliance. By (1) reducing the commands given to those that are important to parents, (2) always providing a consequence, and (3) phrasing commands appropriately, parents can expect to see an increase in their child's compliance.

Before giving a command, the parent should make sure he/she has the child's attention. Saying the child's name, standing in front of the child, and making eye contact are possible ways to establish a connection with the child. Commands should be given one at a time. If a parent would like the child to complete a multistep task, the parent should break the task down into smaller steps. For each step the parent should (1) give a command, (2) wait for the child to comply/not comply, and (3) provide an appropriate consequence. Parents also should make sure that their commands are stated as directives rather than as questions or suggestions. Statements such as "It would be nice if you would clean up your toys" do not tell the child that the toys *must be cleaned up immediately.* If the parent wants this task to be completed, a more appropriate command would be, "Please pick up the toys on your bedroom floor and put them in the toy chest." Commands should be as specific as possible, so that there is no doubt as to what is expected from the child.

If a task involves a choice, parents can include the choice in their command. For example, if a mother is directing her child to put on her shoes—but the child can wear either her sneakers or her boots—the mother might say, "Addie, we're ready to go to the park now. Please put on either your white sneakers or your brown boots." Rationales for commands should be brief and presented either before the command (as in the previous

PLAYTIME HOMEWORK SHEET

Child's name _____

Date	Did you practice? (Yes or No)	Any comments

FIGURE 3.3. Playtime homework sheet. From Gretchen A. Gimpel and Melissa L. Holland (2003). Copyright by The Guilford Press. Permission to photocopy this figure is granted to purchasers of this book for personal use only (see copyright page for details).

example) or after the child complies. For example, after complying with the commands to "Please put on your white sneakers or brown boots," the parent says, "Thank you for putting on your boots as I asked. I wanted to you put on shoes because we're ready to go to the park now." Preschool children do not need lengthy rationales; they often *ask* for rationales (i.e., "why?") simply to delay complying with the command. Particularly with young children, parents should ensure that the child is physically capable of completing any command given (Barkley, 1997; Hembree-Kigin & McNeil, 1995; Schroeder & Gordon, 2002).

These guidelines for giving appropriate commands are discussed in session with parents, and they are given a handout (see Figure 3.4) that summarizes the use of commands. After learning how to give appropriate commands, parents are taught to use specific disciplinary techniques for those occasions of noncompliance. It is very important that parents continue to use the positive skills previously learned as they learn new disciplinary skills. Parents should continue to engage in the structured play activity on a regular basis; in addition, they should learn to be attuned to opportunities throughout the day to positively reinforce their child's behaviors. Parents should always provide positive reinforcement as soon as the child complies with a given command.

The discipline technique of choice with preschool- and kindergarten-age children is time-out. Most parents have had some experience with time-out and often insist that it "does not work" for their child. Thus one of the first tasks a clinician faces is "selling" the parents on the use of a technique they would choose not to use. When time-out does not work it is typically because parents do not use it in an appropriate manner. True time-out involves removing the child from all reinforcers. Many parents continue to talk to their children while they are supposedly in time-out. Although the content of what is said may be negative (e.g., "Sit down. You need to learn to behave or you'll never get out of time-out"), the attention that the child is receiving is typically reinforcing. Thus, in such instances, the child is not truly experiencing a time-out.

Parents often leave their children in time-out for excessively long periods of time. The general rule of thumb is that children should be in time-out 1 minute per year of age, not to exceed 5 minutes. Extensive time-outs can be difficult to enforce, and they deny children learning opportunities. The time-out should be brief so that children can get out of it, engage in negative or positive behaviors, and receive appropriate consequences. Repeated instances of (1) the child performing an inappropriate behavior and being sent to time-out, and (2) the child performing an appropriate behavior and receiving positive reinforcement help the child learn which behaviors are appropriate and which are not. Parents also may believe that time-out does not work because the child will not automatically stay in it. Parents may become frustrated that their child is continually leaving the time-out location and, because they are unsure what to do, they simply let the child end his/her own time-out. In such situations, the child learns he/she can escape with no consequence, and, obviously, time-out becomes ineffective.

Time-out is explained to parents in session, and they are given a handout (see Figure 3.5) on its use. Any information the parents have provided to the clinician about their previous use of time-out should be acknowledged and addressed. Parents are initially taught to use time-out in response to noncompliant behavior. After giving a command (e.g., "Please hand me a tissue."), parents are instructed to wait 10 seconds for the child to com-

GIVING EFFECTIVE COMMANDS

When giving commands to your child, you may be able to improve compliance rates simply by following these guidelines.

1. **Save commands for times you can follow through.** Only give commands in situations in which it is important that a command be given. Make sure you can provide consequences for compliance/noncompliance and always provide consequences.

2. **Get your child's attention.** Prior to giving a command, make sure you have your child's attention. Make eye contact, say your child's name, etc. You should always be in the same room as your child when giving a command, and you should reduce potential distractions (e.g., turn off the TV or stereo).

3. **Only give commands your child is capable of completing.** Tasks involving activities that are too difficult for your child to understand or complete adequately should not be given.

4. **Make commands direct and simple.** Commands should be phrased as statements in a polite, matter-of-fact tone of voice. Do not phrase commands as questions or suggestions.

5. **Give only one command at a time.** Children often have difficulties following through with multiple-step commands. Give one command at a time, with a consequence for compliance/ noncompliance after each command.

6. **State commands positively.** Instead of telling your child what *not* to do ("Don't jump on the bed"), tell your child what *to do* ("Please get off the bed and go outside to play.").

7. **Make limited use of explanations.** Often children ask for explanations or rationales simply to avoid complying with a command. Rationales should be given either before the command ("We're going to visit Grandma, and it's cold outside, so you need to put on your coat now.") or after the child complies with the command ("Please put on your coat [Child complies.] Thank you for putting on your coat. We're walking over to Grandma's and it's cold outside.").

8. **If possible, give choice commands.** If the child can make a choice, let the child know that in the command (e.g., "Please put on your red coat or your blue coat.").

FIGURE 3.4. Giving effective commands. From Gretchen A. Gimpel and Melissa L. Holland (2003). Copyright by The Guilford Press. Permission to photocopy this figure is granted to purchasers of this book for personal use only (see copyright page for details).

EFFECTIVELY USING TIME-OUT

Time-out is an effective method to reduce your child's inappropriate behaviors. However, it should always be used in combination with other techniques you have already learned. Make sure you are positively attending to appropriate behaviors and using effective commands. Never give a command that you do not intend to back up, and always provide praise when your child complies with a command. To effectively use time-out with your child, follow the guidelines below:

1. **Give an appropriate command.** Always give appropriate commands in a firm, neutral voice. (See Giving Effective Commands handout.)

2. **Wait 10 seconds.** After giving a command, wait 10 seconds for your child to comply. To make sure you are waiting the full 10 seconds, you may want to count to yourself—but make sure you do not count out loud. If you count out loud, your child learns he/she does not need to comply until you get to 10.

3. **If no compliance, restate the command and wait 10 seconds.** If your child has not begun to comply within 10 seconds, you should say firmly, "If you don't _____ [repeat the command], then you will go to time-out." After giving this warning, wait another 10 seconds for compliance.

   Note: When you are using time-out for something other than noncompliance (e.g., breaking a set rule), send the child to time-out immediately and do not use this warning statement.

4. **Send/take child to time-out.** If your child has still not started to comply with your command within these 10 seconds, say, "You did not do as I asked, so you must go to time-out." Speak calmly but firmly. Following this statement, the child must go to time-out immediately. The child should not be allowed to argue, belatedly comply with the command, etc. Initially you may need to use physical guidance to get your child to the time-out location. Try gently leading your child by the arm. If necessary, pick up your child from behind and carry him/her to the time-out location. Once the child is in the time-out location, say firmly, "Stay there until I tell you to come out."

5. **Do not attend to the child.** Do not give the child any attention while he/she is in time-out. Do not talk to the child at all. You should go back to doing what you were doing, but make sure to keep an eye on the child (without staring at him/her). When the child has remained in the time-out quietly for the appropriate amount of time (see below), return to the child and say, "You may come out of time-out now."

6. **Restate the command.** After your child is released from time-out, repeat your original command. If the child complies, praise him/her. If the child does not comply, he/she should be sent to time-out again.

7. **Praise appropriate behavior.** Watch for your child's next appropriate behavior and praise him/her for it.

(continued)

FIGURE 3.5. Effectively using time-out. From Gretchen A. Gimpel and Melissa L. Holland (2003). Copyright by The Guilford Press. Permission to photocopy this figure is granted to purchasers of this book for personal use only (see copyright page for details).

FREQUENTLY ASKED QUESTIONS ABOUT TIME-OUT

How Long Should My Child Stay in Time-Out?

The general rule of thumb is that children should remain quiet in time-out for about 1 minute per year of age, not to exceed 5 minutes. However, when initially using time-out, this time frame is typically too much to expect, so plan on working up to it. When time-out is first used, it is common for children to cry, whine, scream, etc., for long periods of time. If this behavior occurs, release your child from time-out once your child has been quiet for a few moments (10–30 seconds). Gradually you can increase the amount of time you require your child to remain quiet.

Where Should My Time-Out Location Be?

For young children, time-out in a chair is the preferable method. The chair should be an adult-size dining-room type chair. It should be placed far enough away from all objects (including walls) that the child cannot kick or hit anything while in the chair. There should be nothing reinforcing that the child has access to from the chair (e.g., TV, radio). The time-out chair should be placed in a location that you can observe (e.g., in a hallway, not in a closet or bathroom).

What If the Child Leaves the Time-Out Chair?

It is not uncommon for children to test the limits when parents first begin to use time-out. Children will often leave the chair and may do so immediately after being placed in time-out. It is important that, if this happens, you immediately return the child to time-out. Each time the child gets out, you should return the child to the chair. The first couple times you return the child, state in a firm, calm voice, "You need to stay in time-out until you are quiet." When first using time-out (when it is most likely the child will leave the chair), it is a good idea to stand right next to the chair (but do not look directly at the child or do anything to give the child attention.) That way, you can immediately put the child back in time-out as soon as he/she leaves the time-out chair. Children who squirm, bounce, roll around, stand, etc., in the chair should not be considered out of time-out. This behavior should simply be ignored.

What Should I Do If My Child Says He/She Needs to Get Out of the Chair?

The child is not to leave the time-out chair to use the bathroom or get a drink until his/her time is up and he/she has completed the task that was asked of him/her. If your child is permitted to leave time-out following a certain demand, he/she will come to use this demand as a means of escaping from time-out on each occasion he/she is placed in the chair. Simply ignore all requests your child makes.

ply. If the child does not comply within that time period, the parent repeats the command and tells the child he/she will go to time-out if he/she does not comply (e.g., "Please hand me a tissue or you will go to time-out."). Again, the child is given 10 seconds to begin to comply. If the child still does not comply, the parent should send the child to time-out (e.g., "You didn't hand me a tissue, as I asked, so you need to go to time-out.").

Of course, most children will not willingly go to time-out, so the parent often will need to lead the child to the time-out location. If the child will not walk with assistance to time-out, the parent should pick up the child from behind and place him/her in time-out, making one brief directive statement such as, "You need to stay there until I tell you to come out." While the child is in the time-out location, all verbalizations and activities are ignored. It is extremely important that the parent understand why he/she should ignore the child during the time-out period—that is, that attending to the child is reinforcing and defeats the purpose. If the child leaves the time-out location, he/she should be placed back in time-out immediately. Initially the parent may have to stand very close to the time-out location so that he/she can return the child to time-out immediately.

When time-out is first used, children can take a long time to quiet down and stop crying. Thus, initially parents may be instructed to let the child out of time-out as soon as he/she is quiet for a very brief period of time (e.g., 10 seconds). Gradually, this time would be increased, so that the child learns to remain quiet for longer periods (i.e., 1 minute per year of age, with a maximum quiet time of 5 minutes). When the child has been quiet for the appropriate length of time, the parent should let the child out of time-out with the explanation "You're being quiet, so you may come out of time-out now.". Once the child is released from time-out, the parent should repeat the original command and provide the appropriate consequence (i.e., praise for compliance, another time-out for noncompliance). It is very important that parents complete this last step of reissuing the original command otherwise children may come to view time-out as a way of escaping something they do not want to do.

The location of the time-out is important to discuss with parents in session. Parents sometimes have difficulty enforcing time-outs because they place the child in locations they cannot see (e.g., at the end of a hallway) or near something the child can reach and destroy (e.g., placing a child near a lamp he/she can reach and knock over). Parents are instructed to use an adult-sized straight-back chair for time-out. (Although using a chair is not the only option, it is typically easier to implement a time-out in a chair initially.) Ideally the child's feet should not reach the floor. The chair should be located so that the parent can see the child, but the child cannot access any potential reinforcers (e.g., the child should not be able to see the TV). In addition, the chair should be located in an area in which there is nothing within arms' or legs' reach of the child.

Although many parents use timers to track the length of time the child is in time-out, the use of a timer can present some problems. When a timer is used, parents and children may come to view the sounding of the timer as an indicator that time-out is over. It is important that it is *the parent* (not the timer) who releases the child from time-out and that the child is let out *once he/she is quiet* (not once the timer sounds). Therefore, if parents use timers, they should make it clear to the child that he/she will not be dismissed from time-out until the parent indicates it is time. Timers are typically most helpful for parents who might "forget" that their child is in time-out. However, given that parents should be taught to monitor their child during time-out so that they can (1) immediately return the child to time-out if the child escapes, and (2) release the child from time-out once the child is quiet, many believe that timers are not needed and may actually create problems for parents.

Because of the potential problems with using time-out, it is extremely helpful if parents have an opportunity to practice it in a therapy session. Once the clinician has explained the use of commands and time-out to the parent, the parent is coached on his/her application of it in session. This phase begins by asking the parent to interact with his/her child in a play context. Gradually the parent begins to give commands to the child. At first these commands should be relatively easy for the child to comply with (e.g., "Please hand me the red block" in reference to a block the child is not currently using), but gradually the parent should make the commands more demanding in an attempt to elicit noncompliance in session (e.g., "Please put the blocks away."). The clinician should coach the parent on his/her use of commands to ensure that the parent is phrasing them appropriately. When the child complies with a command, the parent should always praise the child for compliance (e.g., "Thank you for handing me the red block like I asked you to do."). If the child does not comply, the parent is coached through the process of putting the child in time-out and ignoring him/her for that time period. This component that requires ignoring the child can be very difficult for parents initially. Many young children scream and cry vigorously and may use hurtful words in their attempts to secure their parents' attention (e.g., "You don't really love me," "I hate you").

Once time-out has been covered in session, parents are instructed to begin using it at home, tracking their use of it as well as any problems they encounter (see Figure 3.6). After parents have implemented the use of time-out for noncompliance, the clinician helps the parent identify "house rules" for which the child will receive a time-out if broken. Parents should be encouraged to set a limited number of house rules (two or three is a good number to begin with, for young children) and save these rules for things that are important. When the child fails to follow a house rule, he/she is immediately sent to time-out. No warning is given in this situation.

Additional Reinforcement/Discipline Methods

Although time-out is the discipline method of choice for young children, alternative methods, such as contingency contracting, also may be used. Contingency contracting may involve a comprehensive token economy system, in which poker chips or points (which can be exchanged for tangible reinforcers) are given to the child for appropriate behavior and taken away for inappropriate behavior. However, token economy systems can get quite complex and cumbersome for parents, and a simplified system is often the easier way to go. Using privileges (instead of tokens or points that must be exchanged) can be easier for parents. When using privileges to manage behavior, parents should begin by listing the privileges their child can earn for appropriate behaviors and those that will be taken away for inappropriate behaviors (see Figures 3.7 and 3.8). The privileges that the child can earn by exhibiting positive, prosocial behavior would be extra privileges that the child receives, in

TIME-OUT HOMEWORK SHEET

Child's Name _____

Date	Did you use time out?(Yes or No)	Length of Time-Outs	Problems?

FIGURE 3.6. Time-out homework sheet. From Gretchen A. Gimpel and Melissa L. Holland (2003). Copyright by The Guilford Press. Permission to photocopy this figure is granted to purchasers of this book for personal use only (see copyright page for details).

USING PRIVILEGES TO MANAGE BEHAVIOR

Privileges can be used to reinforce your child for appropriate behaviors and to discipline him/her for inappropriate behaviors. This method may be used when it is not possible to use time-out or as an addition to time-out to reinforce or punish specific behaviors. Below are guidelines to follow when using privileges.

Providing Privileges for Appropriate Behavior

1. With your child, make up a list of privileges he/she can earn. These should include extra-special privileges (e.g., getting a new toy, eating at McDonalds with a parent) as well as other, common privileges (e.g., 15-minute later bedtime, extra dessert, watching an additional TV show).

2. Make a list of behaviors and chores that your child can do to earn privileges. Make sure that you do not place unreasonable expectations on your child. Good examples of chores/tasks for young children are: picking up toys, helping set the table, putting away clean clothes, helping feed the dog, etc.

3. When your child completes a chore or behavior on your list, give him/her one of the privileges, making sure to praise your child for completing the behavior/chore. For example, when your child earns the privilege of watching an extra TV show, you might say, "Thanks for taking your toys out of the living room. Because you did such a good job cleaning up, you may watch 'Barney' and 'Sesame Street' today." Provide your child with the common extra privileges on a regular basis and occasionally give him/her one of the extra-special privileges.

4. Provide lots of reinforcement, especially initially. When beginning the program, look for opportunities to give your child privileges for appropriate behaviors, and remember that you can reward your child for good behaviors that are not on the list you have made. Parents often expect too much at once and wait for "big" behaviors to occur before providing reinforcement. This makes it less likely that the program will be successful, because the child will rarely have access to the privileges.

Taking Away Privileges for Inappropriate Behavior

1. Make a list of privileges your child automatically receives on a daily basis. These privileges are those your child does not need to do anything special to obtain but are the everyday privileges you allow your child (e.g., an hour of television, unlimited access to all toys, inviting a friend over).

2. Make a list of behaviors/chores that your child must do in order to keep these automatic privileges. This list should be relatively short and should include only those chores or tasks that your child is expected to complete on a daily basis (e.g., getting dressed for preschool, brushing teeth at night).

(continued)

FIGURE 3.7. Using privileges to manage behavior. From Gretchen A. Gimpel and Melissa L. Holland (2003). Copyright by The Guilford Press. Permission to photocopy this figure is granted to purchasers of this book for personal use only (see copyright page for details).

3. Make a list of inappropriate behaviors that you will not tolerate from your child (e.g., hitting siblings, spitting out food at the dinner table).

4. As long as your child completes the daily tasks identified in step 2, he/she is allowed to keep his/her automatic privileges. If these daily tasks are not completed, or your child exhibits one of the inappropriate behaviors identified in step 3, then take away certain automatic privileges. It may be easiest to pair each negative behavior with a specific privilege that will be lost. Go over this list with your child so that he/she knows what is expected of him/her and what will happen when he/she does not complete a daily task or engages in an inappropriate behavior.

It is important to understand that you are not bribing your child. Many parents feel that their children should obey house rules simply because it is their responsibility. Remember, though, that you get paid for working at a job. In the same sense, obeying house rules is your child's job, and he/she should be able to earn privileges in the same way you earn a paycheck.

PRIVILEGES WORKSHEET

Earning Privileges for Appropriate Behaviors

Extra/Optional Behaviors and Chores

1. _____
2. _____
3. _____
4. _____
5. _____
6. _____
7. _____
8. _____
9. _____
10. _____

Extra Privileges

1. _____
2. _____
3. _____
4. _____
5. _____
6. _____
7. _____
8. _____
9. _____
10. _____

Special Extra Privileges

1. _____
2. _____
3. _____
4. _____
5. _____

Removal of Privileges for Inappropriate Behaviors

Expected Behaviors and Chores

1. _____
2. _____
3. _____
4. _____
5. _____
6. _____
7. _____
8. _____
9. _____
10. _____

Automatic Privileges

1. _____
2. _____
3. _____
4. _____
5. _____
6. _____
7. _____
8. _____
9. _____
10. _____

Inappropriate Behaviors

1. _____
2. _____
3. _____
4. _____
5. _____

FIGURE 3.8. Privileges worksheet. From Gretchen A. Gimpel and Melissa L. Holland (2003). Copyright by The Guilford Press. Permission to photocopy this figure is granted to purchasers of this book for personal use only (see copyright page for details).

addition to his/her everyday privileges (e.g., watching an hour of TV). The privileges that are removed for inappropriate behaviors would be those everyday privileges that the child automatically receives; when a rule is broken or an expected task not performed, the child loses one of these everyday privileges. Tangible reinforcers can be used in addition to privileges in this system.

Parents also could set up a positive reinforcement system in which a child earns points toward a specific reinforcer. For example, if a child wants to see a certain movie, his/her parents could create a chart that has a picture of a character in this movie at the end of a "road." Each time the child engages in an appropriate behavior, he/she is able to move a marker down the road and one step close to the movie character. When the child's marker reaches the character, he/she earns the reinforcer (i.e., going to the movie). When this method is used with young children, it is important that they be able to earn the reinforcer quickly. If they must wait for several days or weeks, the delay between the behavior and the reinforcer will be too long and the intervention will be unsuccessful.

Generalization and Maintenance of Skills

Initially the skills described above are taught and practiced with the home setting in mind. Obviously, though, it is important that parents learn to generalize these skills to situations outside the home, such as grocery stores, restaurants, department stores, etc. Before attempting to apply the skills outside the home, the clinician should ensure that the parent can easily use the skills in session. Parents who are still struggling with giving appropriate commands or using discipline skills in a consistent manner in the home will have added difficulties applying the skills outside the home. Teaching parents to generalize skills to other settings is typically the last component of parent training. (See Figure 3.9 for the handout explaining this step.)

When parents first practice these new skills outside the home, they should begin with "training trips." These trips should be relatively brief, and it should not be imperative that the parents complete the trip. For example, a parent may take a training trip to the grocery store to pick up just a few items that he/she does not have to obtain that day. Before embarking on this trip, the parent should set up rules with the child. For example, rules for appropriate grocery store behavior might include: (1) Stay within arm's reach of the cart, (2) do not take items off the shelf unless told to do so by mom or dad, and (3) talk in your indoor voice. Once in the store, the parent should make sure to praise the child for following the rules and for any other appropriate behaviors. Parents may want to engage their children in the shopping experience by directing them to take certain items off the shelf and put them in the cart.

Parents also should consider setting up a reward program for complying with the rules. For example, when the child follows the rules or engages in other appropriate behaviors, the parent would give the child a token. If the child has a certain number of tokens by the end of the shopping trip, he/she can exchange the tokens for a reinforcer (e.g., a candy bar, a movie to watch at home). For inappropriate behaviors, parents can use time-out in the store (e.g., they can have the child sit on the floor in an out-of-the-way section of the store), but because many parents feel uncomfortable with this idea, it is often not a viable

MANAGING BEHAVIOR PROBLEMS IN PUBLIC PLACES

After your child has learned to comply with rules and commands at home, it will be easier to teach him/her to behave as expected in public places, such as stores and restaurants. When out in public, it is important to praise appropriate behaviors and provide consequences for inappropriate behaviors, just as you would do at home. Below are guidelines to help you.

1. **Take practice trips.** Take several short trips as trial runs before making a longer trip. Limit these trips to 15–20 minutes and make their sole purpose to practice these guidelines.

2. **Set up rules beforehand.** Before entering the store or other public place, always review with your child the rules you expect him/her to follow. You should have three or four rules. For example, if you are taking your child grocery shopping, your rules might be: "stay within arm's length of the cart, do not take any items off the shelves, and talk in your indoor voice."

3. **Praise your child for good behaviors.** As you have been doing at home, provide your child with positive reinforcement for appropriate behaviors. Make sure to tell your child specifically what you like about his/her behavior, and frequently praise your child when he/she is following the preset rules. You also may want to consider providing some reward for your child—perhaps some special time with you at home following the trip or a special treat at the end of the trip. You may also use a point or token system in which the child is able to earn points/tokens (items that can later be exchanged for special reinforcers) for appropriate behaviors.

4. **Set up consequences for misbehavior.** You must have predetermined consequences you can enforce for misbehaviors. These should be explained to your child. One way to address misbehavior is to use a point system. If you are using a point/token system to reinforce your child for appropriate behaviors, you can add a response cost component in whcih you take away points/tokens for inappropriate behaviors. As an alternative, prior to your trip, give your child a predetermined number of points, which can later be exchanged for some privilege or treat. As your child misbehaves, subtract points from this total. Your child is allowed to "spend" the points he/she still has at the end of the trip. You should determine what the points can be used to buy (i.e., will you allow the child to buy candy, or does the child need to spend the points on a special privilege once at home?).

   You should also consider using time-out in public if you have successfully used this with your child at home. You may use an area of a floor or a seat to the side of a table for this. Remember that time-out does not always have to occur in a chair.

5. **Give your child something to do.** Often children misbehave because they have nothing to do. When you are out in public with your child, talk to him/her frequently and provide small tasks to do. For example, if you are grocery shopping, you might ask your child to reach for the items on the lower shelves (only after you have pointed the items out to the child).

6. **If your child throws a tantrum—*do not give in.*** If your child throws a tantrum in an attempt to get candy or some other treat, do not give in. Ignore your child, if possible, and leave the store, restaurant, etc., if necessary, until your child calms down. (*Note:* Never leave your child alone— you should always accompany your child when it becomes necessary to leave the public place.)

FIGURE 3.9. Managing behavior problems in public places. From Gretchen A. Gimpel and Melissa L. Holland (2003). Copyright by The Guilford Press. Permission to photocopy this figure is granted to purchasers of this book for personal use only (see copyright page for details).

option. Instead, parents can add a response-cost component to the reward system in which the child loses tokens for inappropriate behaviors. If the child begins to throw a tantrum in the store, it is very important that the parent not give in to the behavior, however embarrassing. For example, if the child begins to throw a tantrum because his/her mother will not give him/her the candy he/she wants, it is imperative that the mother not give the child the candy just to stop the tantrum. Doing so would only serve to teach the child that a long enough or loud enough tantrum will get him/her what he/she wants. In this situation the child should be ignored if possible. If this is too difficult for the parent to do, the child should be taken outside the store. It is very important, though, that parents never leave their children unattended. Children should never be taken to the car and simply left there.

In addition to learning how to generalize skills to situations outside the home, parents also need help planning for generalization in situations in which they are not present (e.g., preschool)—especially if their children have problems across settings. The clinician could consult with the preschool teacher (along with the parent) and set up a similar behavior management program in school. Another option would be to use a home–school note system (e.g., Kelley, 1990; described in more detail later in this chapter).

Ensuring that skills are maintained over time is also obviously important. Unfortunately, there is little empirical research regarding the best way to promote maintenance of treatment gains (Eyberg, Edwards, Boggs, & Foote, 1998). One option often used is to provide "booster sessions" for parents. Such sessions might involve brief (e.g., 30 minutes to an hour) monthly meetings, wherein skills are reviewed and practiced and any problem areas discussed.

Group Parent Training

Conducting parent training in a group setting is an option clinicians may want to consider if they do not have the time or resources to implement individual parent training. Group parent training is conducted in the same manner as the individualized format. However, the child is typically not present and the parents do not have the opportunity to practice skills in session with their children. Instead, the parents typically engage in role playing with other parents and then practice the skills at home with their children. Because children are not present, group parent training programs often make use of videotaped models so that parents can see the application of the skills with actual children.

Probably the best known and most researched group behavioral parent training program is Carolyn Webster-Stratton's videotape-based program. Data from her studies indicate that this program is effective and that parents like it (Webster-Stratton, 1984, 1994; Webster-Stratton & Hammond, 1997). In this program, the same basic format discussed above is followed. Parents are taught to attend to their children's positive behaviors, then they are taught to use effective commands and time-out for inappropriate behaviors. Skills are modeled in session through the use of videotaped vignettes, and parents role play the skills with one another. The vignettes depict parents modeling both the appropriate and inappropriate use of the skills, which allows for discussion among the participants on what components are involved in the appropriate use of the skills. The use of these models seems to be a key component in the program: Webster-Stratton has noted superior effects of her program when the videotaped models are used than when they are not used (Webster-Stratton & Hancock, 1998).

In addition to the basic parent training program, Webster- Stratton has developed an add-on program specifically to address parents' needs. Sessions focus on issues such as communication, anger management, and problem solving. In addition, parents are taught how to assist their children in learning problem-solving skills. These add-on sessions have been found to provide benefits to parents in the targeted areas (e.g., improved communication) above those obtained in a parent-training–only intervention; however, there were no differences in improvement in child behavior problems (Webster-Stratton, 1994).

Group parent training seems to be as effective as individual parent training (Serketich & Dumas, 1996; Webster-Stratton, 1984) and is clearly more cost-effective (e.g., Webster-Stratton, 1984). However, there are some potential disadvantages to using the group format. Although parents in a group may benefit from sharing knowledge and experience with one another, this format and the sharing are uncomfortable for some parents. In addition, parents whose skills are very lacking may need more individualized attention than can be provided in a group setting. Individual parent training allows the clinician to address the specific needs of the family and to pace the treatment program so that it is most appropriate for the family.

PRESCHOOL- AND KINDERGARTEN-BASED BEHAVIORAL INTERVENTION PROGRAMS

With young children increasingly attending daycare and preschool facilities, clinicians who work with this population need to have skills in setting up school-based programs as well as home-based ones. The same techniques used in the home setting can also be applied to the school setting. As with home-based interventions, the key to effective school-based interventions for disruptive behavior problems is providing positive reinforcement for appropriate behaviors and using mild punishment for inappropriate behaviors. Specific techniques that may be used in the school (or daycare) setting are reviewed below. A summary of these techniques is provided in Table 3.2.

One of the most important elements in a classroom is a posted list of rules. These rules should clearly communicate to the students what behaviors are expected and considered

TABLE 3.2. Summary of Classroom
Intervention Techniques

Posting of rules
Selective attention/verbal praise
Token reinforcement system
Response cost (e.g., removal of tokens)
Time-out
Classwide programs
Home–school notes

appropriate in the classroom setting. Rules should be kept to a minimum so as to not over-whelm the teacher or the students, and they should be focused on the most important aspects of classroom behavior. Rules should be stated in a positive manner that tells the students what *to do* rather than what *not* to do. For example, instead of posting "No run-ning in the hallway," the rule might be worded: "Always walk in the hallway." Rules should be posted (with pictorial reminders for nonreaders) and reviewed with the class periodi-cally. Rules that may be appropriate to the preschool classroom include: "Keep hands and feet to self" and "Stay seated during teacher-directed activities."

Teachers should use selective attention on a regular basis to reinforce their students for appropriate, on-task behaviors. When the teacher notices a child is following a class-room rule or otherwise behaving appropriately, the teacher should deliver a brief, labeled praise statement (e.g., "Jennifer, I like how you're sitting in your seat and listening to my instructions."). In addition to using praise, teachers also can use a token reinforcement sys-tem to increase the likelihood of appropriate behaviors. When the teacher sees a child engaging in an appropriate behavior, the teacher gives the student a token (e.g., poker chip, a star on a chart) accompanied by a brief praise statement. If the child has earned a certain number of tokens by the end of the school day, he/she is able to exchange them for a tangible reinforcer (e.g., stickers, small toys). Although there are some behaviors teachers must discipline, they can ignore minor, annoying behaviors and instead reinforce whatever appropriate behavior is exhibited. For example, if a child is playing with toys rambunc-tiously (but not in a destructive manner), the teacher may want to ignore this behavior while praising a child who is playing appropriately (e.g., "Tony, I really like how you're building nicely with the Legos.").

Although it is always important to have positive consequences in place for appropriate behaviors, adding a response-cost component may increase the efficacy of classroom-based interventions. Studies with school-age children who have ADHD have shown that provid-ing only positive reinforcement for appropriate behaviors is not enough to change behavior on a consistent basis (e.g., Sullivan & O'Leary, 1990). Instead, a response-cost program, in which children lose positives for inappropriate behavior, is also needed. This finding also may apply to preschool-age children (McGoey & DuPaul, 2000). In addition, utilizing a response-cost program may be more acceptable to teachers, because it may be easier to implement than a positive-reinforcement–only program, in which teachers must be con-stantly looking for instances of appropriate behaviors to reinforce (McGoey & DuPaul). In a response-cost system, each child begins the day with a certain number of tokens. When a child breaks a classroom rule or engages in another inappropriate behavior, the teacher notes which classroom rule the child broke and takes away a token. At the end of the day, each child is able to exchange remaining tokens (if any) for a tangible reinforcer.

In one successful response-cost program in the preschool classroom, children were given cards with laminated smiley-faces attached to them with velcro. Each time a child engaged in an inappropriate behavior, a smiley face was removed from the card. Children who still had smiley faces on their cards at the end of the observation period were allowed to choose a reward from a reward menu. At the end of the week, children who had earned a smiley face at least 4 of the days were allowed to draw from a grab bag that contained a variety of small toys (Reynolds & Kelley, 1997). In another preschool classroom-based response-cost system, buttons placed on a chart were used as tokens. Children started each classroom activity (10–15 minutes in duration) with five small buttons and one big button. When a child broke a rule, one of his/her small buttons was removed from the chart. If the child had at least three buttons at the end of the activity, he/she was allowed to keep the big button. At the end of the day, children who had at least three big buttons earned a tangible reward (McGoey & DuPaul, 2000).

Although reinforcement and response-cost systems can be used alone sometimes, teachers can also combine the two. In such a system, children would earn tokens for appropriate behavior (as in the token reinforcement program) and lose them for inappropriate behavior (as in the response-cost system). For token systems to work effectively, children must be able to exchange their tokens on a regular basis for tangible reinforcers. For younger children, this exchange should occur on a daily basis, at least when the program is initiated. It is also important that these tangible reinforcers vary, so that the children do not become bored and disinterested. For example, if students receive stickers every day they have a certain number of tokens remaining, eventually they will become tired of the stickers and the stickers will lose their reinforcing properties. Allowing children to choose from a variety of rewards (e.g., stickers, small toys, special privileges) will help objects maintain their reinforcing value.

In addition to utilizing a token program based on individual performance, teachers may also want to consider implementing a classroom-wide behavior management program, such as the Good Behavior Game (Barrish, Saunders, & Wolf, 1969). In this "game" the class is divided into two teams. Every time a child breaks a classroom rule or engages in an inappropriate behavior, a mark is made for that child's team. The team with the lowest number of points "wins," but both teams can earn reinforcers or special privileges if the number of marks received is below a certain amount. There are a number of variations on this group contingency program. For example, rather than receive marks for inappropriate behaviors, teams could earn points for appropriate behaviors, or a combination of the two may be implemented. In addition, rather than splitting the class into teams, the class as a whole could work toward a reinforcer. When working with young children, it is helpful to use pictures or simple charts so that students can see how many more points they still need to earn a reinforcer. Pfiffner and Barkley (1998) suggest displaying a poster depicting the reward to be earned; when the team (or class as a whole) earns a point, a figure on the poster is moved closer to the picture of the reinforcer.

In addition to token systems, time-out is sometimes used in the classroom. Although teachers are often reluctant to implement time-out, and there are some ethical issues to consider (e.g., excluding children from the classroom; potential to use ineffectively by leaving the child in time-out for long periods of time), it can be used effectively in preschool classrooms. Turner and Watson (1999) provide an overview of the use of time-out in the preschool classroom. Because efforts should be made to keep children in the classroom, it is recommended that an isolation time-out in which the child is removed from the classroom not be used. Time-outs in which the child is removed from the current activity but not the classroom setting are considered to be the most appropriate. Such time-outs may involve complete exclusion, in which the child cannot participate in or view the activity, or partial exclusion, in which the child is removed from the activity but can still view it.

If time-out is to be used in the classroom, the teacher should first explain it to the children. This explanation should be kept brief with young children, but it also should be clear that when a child misbehaves (as defined by existing classroom rules), then the child will be sent to time-out. The teacher should model for the students what is involved in time-out and how one must behave to be allowed out of time-out. As when time-out is applied at home, it should be used consistently when children do not follow the classroom rules. At times this may involve stopping ongoing teaching in order to place a child in time-out (Turner & Watson, 1999). Obviously, implementing this method is easier with at least two adults in the classroom; if an aide is present, they should both follow the same guidelines for time-out use and consider forming an agreement on who does what to implement time-out.

The time-out location selected in the classroom should be a place where the child is removed from ongoing activity but can be easily monitored by the teacher or aide. Time-out should not last for extensively long periods of time. The "1 minute per year of age, not to exceed 5 minutes" guideline is appropriate for classroom time-outs as well as home time-outs. If a child repeatedly attempts to leave the time-out location, he/she should be returned to it. This will only work, realistically, if an aide (or other second adult) is present in the classroom. Teachers working alone may want to reconsider using time-out in the classroom. A barrier to keep the child in time-out also may be used, but this solution has logistical and equipment problems (e.g., what will be used for a barrier) that make it less than ideal (Turner & Watson, 1999).

Home–school notes (mentioned above), which are used commonly with school-age children, can also be implemented with preschool children. The purpose of the home–school note is to enhance communication between the parents and the school while developing contingencies for school-based behaviors. In a typical home–school note system, the teacher evaluates the child on certain behaviors (e.g., raises hand before speaking) throughout the day, and the note is then taken home to the parents—who provide consequences for appropriate or inappropriate behavior (Kelley, 1990). When developing a home–school note, it is important that it be manageable for everyone involved. This means that the note cannot be overly time consuming or complicated. The most salient behaviors should be targeted first. Thus, if the child is having difficulties in play settings due to inappropriate sharing skills, one behavior to include on the home–school note might be "shares with other children during playtime." The behaviors included on the note should be behaviors that can be easily observed by the teacher, and they should be stated in positive terms.

The actual design of home–school notes can vary a great deal. An example of one such note is displayed in Figure 3.10. In this version, the day is divided into time categories. Activity categories (e.g., circle time, recess, lunch) also can be used. Three target behaviors are listed down the side of the note. The teacher then checks "Yes" or "No" for each behavior during each time period to indicate whether the child performed the target behaviors. When teachers are marking the note, they also should provide the child with feedback. For example, the teacher might say, "Joel, you did a great job sharing your toys and following directions, but you still need to work on keeping your hands and feet to yourself."

Instead of a Yes/No system a rating system (e.g., 1–3, where 1 = never, 2 = sometimes, and 3 = always) could be used or, with preschool children, smiley/frowny faces are

SAMPLE HOME–SCHOOL NOTE

Name: _____

	9 A.M.–10 A.M.		10 A.M.–11 A.M.		11 A.M.–12 P.M.		12 P.M.–1 P.M.		1 P.M.–2 P.M.	
	Yes	No	Yes	No	Yes	No	Yes	No	Yes	No
Shares toys										
Keeps hands and feet to self										
Follows directions										

15 points possible;

10 points needed for reward

FIGURE 3.10. Sample home–school note. From Gretchen A. Gimpel and Melissa L. Holland (2003). Copyright by The Guilford Press. Permission to photocopy this figure is granted to purchasers of this book for personal use only (see copyright page for details).

effective. A criterion is set for how many "points" (in the Figure 3.10 example, how many "Yes" marks) a child needs to receive in order to obtain a reward at home. It is important that this number be relatively low at first so that the child is able to succeed. Over time, the number of points needed for a reward can be increased. It is extremely important that parents follow through with providing the reward at home, when the child receives the needed number of points. It is also important that the home–school note actually make it home. For school-age children, a response-cost system is often included so that the child loses certain privileges for that evening if he/she does not bring the note home (or receives an extremely low number of points). With preschool- and kindergarten-age children, teachers are likely to need to be slightly more proactive in making sure the note reaches the parents. Teachers may put the notes in the folders or backpacks that go home on a daily basis. Parents also should be proactive in asking for the note when the child arrives home. Parents should praise the child liberally if his/her goal has been met for the day and then give the child the earned reinforcer as soon as possible. In some situations the reinforcer may not be appropriate immediately (e.g., the child earned a special dessert following dinner), but the parent should praise the child and mention the reinforcer to come later. As children improve on certain behaviors, these behaviors may be removed from the note and new behaviors targeted.

SOCIAL SKILLS INTERVENTIONS

It is often during the preschool years that social problems develop or first become apparent. Two general types of approaches have been used to teach social skills and social competence to children. The *structured learning approach* to teaching social skills focuses on the step by step teaching of actual skills (e.g., how to start a conversation). The *social problem-solving approach* focuses more on teaching problem-solving skills that can be applied in social situations (e.g., deciding on an appropriate course of action when feeling left out of a playground game).

There are a variety of social skills programs that use the structured learning method of training, all of which involve the following components: (1) introducing and defining the skill through didactic means; (2) modeling the skill; (3) overseeing student rehearsal of the skill; and (4) providing performance feedback on how effectively the student performed the skill in the rehearsal/role play. Programs that use this method are based on a group training format. Small pull-out groups of four to eight children or the whole class of students can participate in a social skills training session. With young children, in particular, it is often recommended that the classroom approach be used. For example, in the popular Skillstreaming program, the authors recommend that training take place in the classroom as well as in other locations in which social skills are important (e.g., playground, lunchroom; McGinnis & Goldstein, 1990). One of the difficulties with teaching social skills is the lack of generalization that occurs from the training setting to real-life settings. Utilizing a classroom approach, in which the teacher is one of the trainers, allows for reinforcement of appropriate social skills throughout the day (not just during the training setting), which is considered to be a key component to promoting generalization and maintenance of the social skills.

In the first step of teaching social skills through a structured learning approach—introducing and defining the skill—the skill is described to the children. Typically the skill is described both generally and in terms of the steps involved in completing it. For example, the skill of following directions, as defined by the Skillstreaming program (McGinnis & Goldstein, 1990), includes the following steps: (1) listen, (2) think about it, (3) ask, if needed, and (4) do it (p. 124). After teaching these steps to the students, the skill is modeled by the group leader so that the children can see how the skill is actually performed. Children then take turns practicing the skill through role plays and receiving feedback from peers and group leaders. Children receive positive reinforcement for appropriate use of the skill and corrective feedback for inappropriate use. Following the session, children are assigned homework to practice the skill in real-life settings.

Because children often do not use the skill appropriately at first, it is important that they receive feedback from parents and teachers. If social skills are taught in a pull-out group format, the teacher should be kept apprised of the skills the children are learning so that he/she can assist with the training in real-life settings. In addition, parents should be involved via homework sheets the child brings home and shares or ongoing contact with the group leaders.

In addition to following these steps, it is important to establish basic group rules and behavioral contingencies for appropriate and inappropriate behavior during group meetings. For example, children who are actively participating should earn points or tokens that can then be exchanged for tangible reinforcers at the end of the group. If children are talking out of turn or engaging in aggressive behavior during the groups, they should lose points or tokens.

Problem-solving skills training is the other main type of intervention that has been used with children to attempt to decrease aggressive behaviors and increase prosocial behaviors. Such programs teach children to go through a series of problem-solving steps when they are faced with a problem (see Table 3.3). Children are first taught to define the problem (e.g., wanting to play with others on the playground but not knowing how to approach them). Next children are taught to identify multiple solutions to the problem. At this stage, the focus is purely on identifying as many solutions as possible, and these solutions will typically include prosocial as well as antisocial solutions. Solutions children may

TABLE 3.3. Problem-Solving Steps

What is the problem?
What are possible solutions to the problem?
What would happen if . . . ? [Evaluate outcomes of each possible solution.]
Which option should I choose?
How did my chosen option work out?

generate in response to the problem of wanting to join a group on the playground include asking to join in, throwing a ball at the group, and asking the teacher to tell them to let other kids play too. After such a list of solutions has been generated, each solution is evaluated (e.g., "If I have the teacher ask if I can play too, the other kids might think I'm a teacher's pet.") and the most appropriate solution is chosen and implemented. Following the implementation of the solution, the child evaluates the outcome of applying an appropriate solution (e.g., "I was scared to ask at first, but they said 'sure,' so it was great.").

Problem-solving programs have had some positive effects for older children, both as solo interventions and in combination with other approaches. For example, Kazdin, Siegel, and Bass (1992) evaluated problem-solving skills training, parent training, and the combination of the two with children ages 7–13 and, in general, found that the combined intervention yielded more positive outcomes than either intervention alone. Research on the use of problem-solving skills with young children, however, is still limited. In a study with preschoolers that compared a child intervention (using problem-solving skills training), parent training, a combination of the two, and no treatment, there were positive effects for the child treatment component. Although the interventions involving parent training produced greater positive changes in child behavior problems, the child-focused intervention did lead to better problem-solving skills for the children and fewer negative peer interactions (Webster-Stratton & Hammond, 1997).

This lack of research on social skills programs targeted to young children is not unique to the problem-solving approach. Although some social skills programs have been developed specifically for preschool-age children (e.g, the preschool version of the Skill-streaming program), much of the outcome research with young children has focused on children with developmental delays rather than on typically developing children. In general, the outcome literature on social skills training is not extremely positive. A particular problem with social skills interventions is that of generalization. Often there is little attempt to generalize skills to situations outside of the small group setting. Unfortunately, even when there is a generalization component to the training, skills still may not generalize (DuPaul & Eckert, 1994). As mentioned above, generalization is probably most likely to occur when the skills are taught in real-life settings.

PREVENTION/EARLY INTERVENTION PROGRAMS

As noted in Chapter 1, many of the preschool children who exhibit externalizing symptoms will continue to display problem behaviors through childhood and adolescence. A large number of these children and their families never receive intervention services, and it is likely that problems exhibited by these children will continue to escalate without intervention. Some of these families will eventually receive services, but these services may come too late. One of the key elements in reducing conduct problems is prevention or early intervention. The longer a child/family goes without treatment, the more difficult it becomes to make meaningful changes. Over the past several years, several large-scale studies have been conducted on prevention/early intervention programs for children with externalizing behavior problems. These prevention programs involve multiple interventions across multiple settings, combining many of the interventions already reviewed into a comprehensive package. These programs typically target parenting skills (through parent training), child social competence (through social skills/social competence training), and general aggressive/disruptive behaviors (through home- and school-based behavioral interventions). Other risk factors associated with conduct problems in children, such as poor academic skills, are also sometimes targeted. Because each of the main intervention components has been described in this chapter, we have not outlined a prevention program, per se, instead choosing to briefly review the literature on some of the existing prevention programs.

A prevention/early intervention program for boys identified as being disruptive in kindergarten was implemented in Montreal by Tremblay and colleagues (Tremblay, Pagani-Kurtz, Masse, Vitaro, & Pihl, 1995). The program consisted of parent training plus social skills training (including problem-solving training) over the course of 2 years (from ages 7–9). These boys were then followed to age 15, evaluated on a yearly basis, and compared to a control group of boys who had not received the prevention program. Although there were some positive benefits to the prevention program early on (higher rate of placement in age-appropriate regular classrooms; a trend toward lower teacher-reported disruptive behavior), the treatment and control groups were equivalent on these variables at the last follow-up. However, the treatment group did self-report lower levels of delinquency. This study highlights the importance of long-term follow-up in evaluating the results of prevention programs.

The Fast Track program is another comprehensive early intervention/prevention program that incorporates parent-focused treatment, classroom interventions, and child-focused interventions. In this program, all children at targeted schools were provided with a classwide intervention that included training in emotional understanding, friendship skills, self-control skills, and social problem-solving skills. In addition, for children identified as "high risk," parenting interventions, social skills training, and academic tutoring were offered. In an evaluation of the program after the first year (at the end of grade 1), some significant positive effects were noted for the high-risk students (e.g., increased social problem solving, increased positive peer interactions, decreased parental physical punishment). However, on many of the variables related to disruptive behavior (e.g., CBCL and TRF externalizing scores), there were no significant improvements (Conduct Problems Prevention Research Group, 1999a). For the non-high-risk children who received the classroom prevention component, significant positive effects were reported for peer-rated aggression and hyperactive–disruptive behavior, and intervention classrooms were rated as more positive. However, there was no improvement in teacher ratings of child behaviors (Conduct Problems Prevention Research Group, 1999b).

Barkley and colleagues recently compared a comprehensive school-based early intervention program to a home-based program and a combined (school and home intervention) program. Children who participated were identified prior to kindergarten entry as having high levels of disruptive behaviors. The comprehensive school-based treatment program included social skills training (incorporating structured learning of social skills, following the Skillstreaming model, and self-control and anger-control training); a classroom token system, including a response-cost component; and other behavioral contingency interventions. The home intervention was a standard 10-week group parent training program. Outcomes indicated that the school-based interventions were effective and led to improvements in children's disruptive behaviors, social skills, and self-control, whereas parent training was not effective. The authors attribute the lack of significant results for the parent training, at least in part, to the fact that a large percentage of parents did not attend many of the parent training sessions (the average number of sessions attended was 30%) and that these parents did not actively seek out services (Barkley et al., 2000). Although the school-based program was initially beneficial, these gains were not maintained at a 2-year follow-up (Shelton et al., 2000).

Webster-Stratton, who has examined group parent training extensively, has recently extended the application of this program from one of intervention to one of prevention. A recent study (Webster-Stratton, 1998) demonstrated the efficacy of an abbreviated videotape-based group parent training program as a prevention method. This program was offered to parents of Head Start children, regardless of the behavior problem status of their children. Results indicated improvement in functioning for all children, with particularly notable changes in those with high levels of behavior problems. More recently, Webster-Stratton and her colleagues have incorporated a school-based intervention component with the parent training component. In this prevention program, parents were given 12 weeks of group parent training that utilized videotaped modeling. In addition, parents received later booster sessions to assist with the transition from Head Start to kindergarten. Head Start teachers received six 1-day inservice trainings over a 6-month period. Teachers were instructed in the use of positive management and appropriate discipline techniques. Teachers also helped aggressive children use problem-solving strategies to reduce negative peer interactions. Results from this study indicated positive effects for children, both at home and at school. There was a significant decrease in child behavior problems at school, and for those parents who attended six or more sessions, a significant decrease in home problems. In addition, parents demonstrated more positive parenting behaviors, and teachers exhibited better classroom management practices. These gains were maintained at a 1-year follow-up with the parents (Webster-Stratton, Reid, & Hammond, 2001).

As can be seen from the results of these prevention/early intervention programs, it can be difficult to produce and maintain positive outcomes. Child conduct problems are seen as some of the most intractable problems of childhood, and these studies illustrate that intractability. However, there were some positive outcomes in all studies. As more research is conducted on conduct problems and their treatment and prevention, it is hoped that specific skills as well as program process variables (e.g., parental involvement) will be identified that will clearly lead to more positive and enduring outcomes.

CHAPTER SUMMARY

This chapter has presented an overview of the more common and empirically supported techniques for working with preschool- and kindergarten-age children who demonstrate externalizing behavior problems. Because of the potential for long-term adverse outcomes for these children, it is important to identify them early on and implement appropriate interventions. By far the intervention with the most support for behavior problems is parent training. Thus this intervention should be considered when any child presents with consistently disruptive behaviors. However, as some recent studies have shown, combining multiple interventions to target functioning across settings may produce a wider array of positive outcomes. Clinicians should consider using a multifaceted intervention that targets the child's behavior both at home and in school/daycare.

4

Treatment of Internalizing Problems

Internalizing disorders are characterized by a wide spectrum of symptoms, including depression, anxiety, somatic complaints, and social isolation. These disorders are often more difficult to detect than overt behavior disorders, particularly in young children. Due to the complexities involved in both the detection and treatment of these symptoms, internalizing problems are often misdiagnosed and left untreated. In addition, young children with anxiety or depression often have a different symptom presentation than do older children, so it is important that clinicians working with young children be aware of these differences. This chapter provides an overview of common symptom presentations as well as prevention and intervention methods for young children with anxiety, depression, and selective mutism.

OVERVIEW OF COMMON FEARS, PHOBIAS, AND ANXIETIES

Fear is a normal response to a perceived threat that may be real or imagined. The emotional response of fear is comprised of *psychological discomfort*, such as worry, anxiety, apprehension, or horror, and *physical arousal*, such as increased heart rate, perspiration, and blood pressure. The feeling of fear is generally a protective and adaptive response that alerts the person to danger and thereby helps him/her to survive.

Fears are a normal part of childhood development as children learn to anticipate danger. The anticipation of danger arouses fear and motivates the child to be cautious, thereby preventing the child from being harmed. For example, children who have learned the potential danger of accepting rides or going places with strangers will likely be more cautious when approached by a stranger, taking steps to ensure their own safety, such as not speaking with the stranger, escaping the situation, and getting help from a trusted adult. The fear most children experience when approached by an adult they do not know is only enough to produce cautious behavior and is therefore adaptive. Children who do not anticipate any danger when approached by a stranger may find themselves in a very perilous situation, such as being kidnapped after accepting a ride from a stranger. However, intense fear, anxiety, or a phobic response to public places or being in situations with unknown people would not be adaptive for a child. Thus it is not necessarily the feeling of fear itself that is problematic but the severity of the fear and the situations in which the fear is experienced.

Children's learning histories will impact how they perceive events in their environments. In a certain situation, one child may perceive him/herself to be threatened (experience fear), whereas another child in the same situation may not. This phenomenon is likely explained by each child's pattern of prior beliefs, emotions, and behaviors, which assists him/her in making a quick determination if danger is or is not present. This skill is adaptive; without it, people would not be able to evaluate situations and make decisions quickly and possibly would remain in the dangerous situations. Though each child's fears will differ somewhat from another child's, particular fears seem to cluster at certain ages (Knell, 2000). Fears commonly seen in infancy typically occur as a reaction to the environment, such as fear in response to loud noises or sudden and unpredictable stimuli. Toddlers tend to have fears surrounding strangers, loud noises, separation from caretakers, novel stimuli, and toileting activities. In the preschool and kindergarten years, fears broaden, often involving the dark, animals, imagined supernatural figures, particular objects, events, and people (Jersild, 1968; Morris & Kratochwill, 1998). In addition, preschool- and kindergarten-age children tend to be fearful of parental separation and abandonment, particularly if they are going to daycare or school for the first time. Elementary school-age children tend to have fears involving natural phenomenon, such as earthquakes and storms, as well as fears related to school, health, and home events. In adolescence, fears often center around personal adequacy, physical illness, economic and political events, peers, and sexual matters (Morris & Kratochwill, 1998). In addition to changes in types of fears over time, the number of fears exhibited tends to decline with age. At all ages, females report more fears than do males (Albano et al., 2003).

There are also age differences in how children express symptoms associated with fear and anxiety. Somatic complaints, including headaches and stomachaches, are commonly seen in preschool- and kindergarten-age children. Whereas older children might talk about feelings of anxiety and distressing thoughts, younger children more often act out their anxiety through excessive and uncontrollable crying, anger outbursts, tantrums, or clinginess (American Psychiatric Association, 1994). In addition, children who have experienced some form of trauma, such as abuse, may express their anxiety through repetitive play, a symptom commonly seen in children with post-traumatic stress disorder (see Chapter 6).

The terms *fear* and *anxiety* are often used interchangeably; however, there are differences between the two. Fear is typically conceptualized as a set of intense physiological responses (e.g., increased heart rate, sweating, shaking) in response to a specific stimuli. For example, a child who is approached by a stranger who attempts to take the child into his/her car would experience fear. Anxiety is considered to be somewhat vaguer and more diffuse and is typically not a response to a specific stimulus. For example, the child who was approached by the stranger may begin to feel tense and apprehensive about being away from his/her parents, even when there is no direct threat (Barrios & O'Dell, 1998).

Specific Phobia

Whereas fears are typical, extreme fears or phobias—in which the fear/phobia is persistent and more severe than would be expected for the age and developmental level of the child—are not as common and may warrant intervention. To determine whether or not a fear has developed into a phobia, several important points must be considered. First, is the fear excessive or unreasonable? Because young children typically cannot determine if their fears are excessive, this judgment will likely be made by the adults in the child's life. Second, does exposure to the situation almost invariably provoke an immediate anxiety response, such as crying, throwing a tantrum, becoming immobilized, or clinging? Third, is the situation or stimulus either avoided or endured only with intense anxiety? Fourth, does the anxiety persist over an extended period of time (American Psychiatric Association, 1994)? The answers to these questions can aid the clinician in determining whether the child's symptoms are indicative of an anxiety disorder and whether treatment is warranted.

A specific phobia involves a marked and persistent fear of clearly discernible, circumscribed objects or situations. Upon exposure to the object/situation, the child experiences an anxiety response; the feared object is often avoided to prevent the anxiety response. In order to be diagnosed with a specific phobia, children do not need to recognize that their fear of the object or situation is excessive (American Psychiatric Association, 1994). Although fears are common in young children, specific, diagnosable phobias are less common. As described previously, fears are typically considered developmentally normal unless the response is much more severe than would be expected in a given situation.

Separation Anxiety

Specific to children, particularly younger children, is anxiety surrounding separation from primary caregivers. When this anxiety is excessive, the child might receive a diagnosis of separation anxiety disorder, (American Psychiatric Association, 1994). Children with this disorder exhibit developmentally excessive anxiety regarding separation from home or attachment figures. At least three of the following must be present and must have occurred for at least 4 weeks for a child to receive this diagnosis (American Psychiatric Association, 1994, p. 113):

(1) recurrent excessive distress when separation from home or major attachment figures occurs or is anticipated
(2) persistent and excessive worry about losing, or about possible harm befalling, major attachment figures
(3) persistent and excessive worry that an untoward event will lead to separation from a major attachment figure (e.g, getting lost or being kidnapped)
(4) persistent reluctance or refusal to go to school or elsewhere because of fear of separation
(5) persistently and excessively fearful or reluctant to be alone or without major attachment figures at home or without significant adults in other settings
(6) persistent reluctance or refusal to go to sleep without being near a major attachment figure or to sleep away from home

(7) repeated nightmares involving the theme of separation
(8) repeated complaints of physical symptoms (such as headaches, stomachaches, nausea, or vomiting) when separation from major attachment figures occurs or is anticipated

Posttraumatic Stress Disorder

Posttraumatic stress disorder (PTSD) is also an anxiety disorder. Although the definition of PTSD is reviewed here, treatment is covered in Chapter 6 because PTSD in young children often emerges as a result of abuse. PTSD occurs after exposure to a traumatic event in which both of the following were present: (1) the child "experienced, witnessed, or was confronted with an event or events that involved actual or threatened death or serious injury, or a threat to the physical integrity of self or others"; and (2) the child's "response involved intense fear, helplessness, or horror" (American Psychiatric Association, 1994, pp. 427–428). In younger children, this second criteria may be expressed through disorganized or agitated behavior. In addition, the traumatic event is persistently reexperienced in one or more of the following ways (American Psychiatric Association, 1994, p. 428):

(1) recurrent or intrusive recollections of the event [which may be expressed through repetitive play in young children]
(2) recurrent distressing dreams of the event [in children, these dreams may not have recognizable content]
(3) acting or feeling as if the traumatic event were recurring [with trauma-specific reenactment possibly occurring in younger children]
(4) intense psychological distress at exposure to internal or external cues that symbolize or resemble an aspect of the event
(5) physiological reactivity on exposure to internal or external cues that symbolize or resemble an aspect of the event

Attempts are made to avoid thoughts, feelings, conversations, activities, people, or places associated with the trauma. In addition, feelings of detachment or inability to recall important aspects of the trauma may be present. Persistent symptoms of increased arousal, such as difficulties sleeping, anger outbursts or irritability, difficulties concentrating, and hypervigilance and exaggerated startle responses also must be exhibited in order to meet criteria for a diagnosis of PTSD (American Psychiatric Association, 1994).

TREATMENT OF ANXIETY PROBLEMS IN YOUNG CHILDREN

Minimizing a child's fears and anxieties by telling him/her that they are "silly" or "stupid" is countertherapeutic. Instead validate the child's feelings by letting him/her know that you understand how upsetting the worries are for him/her and that you would like to help him/her to feel better. Although there may be a tendency to assume that a child's anxiety will dissipate by itself, or that the child is just being "difficult" or "attention seeking," there is evidence that some anxiety problems can persist from early childhood into later childhood and even into adulthood (Huberty, 1998). Thus if a child's fears or worries have become extreme and/or more intense than is expected, it is important that interventions be implemented.

Once an anxiety problem has been identified and the specific symptoms have been defined through an assessment (see Chapter 2), a treatment plan can be developed. Different disorders and symptom constellations often call for similar, though uniquely different, interventions. Outlined here are treatment plans and interventions for common anxiety problems in young children, including specific phobias and separation anxiety.

Specific Phobia

As outlined previously, a phobia is a marked and persistent fear of an object or situation that is out of proportion to what the child's response would be under normal circumstances. It is important to determine (1) if the child's fears are age appropriate (i.e, if they are similar to what other children his/her age experience when confronted with the object or situation), (2) if the object or situation is actively avoided or endured with intense anxiety, and (3) if the anxiety is interfering with the child's normal routine, such as daycare, school, or social functioning, or if there is marked distress about having the phobia (American Psychiatric Association, 1994).

Prevention of Specific Phobias

Steps can be taken that may help prevent childhood fears from escalating into phobic responses. As mentioned above, it is important to avoid belittling the child's fear in a misguided attempt to reduce it. Statements such as "That is ridiculous, there are no monsters outside of your window" may only make the child feel that he/she cannot talk with adults about the fear—a far cry from depotentiating the fear, as was intended. A better approach is to validate the child's fear without confirming that the fear is real. For example, a parent might state, "I understand that the trees make scary shadows outside of your window and that you feel afraid. I know that you know those are just trees outside, but they do move around a lot at night, don't they?" Such a response allows the child to feel understood while, at the same time, helping him/her to make sense of the stimulus that is causing the fear (Garber, Garber, & Spizman, 1992).

Though it is important to avoid belittling the child's fear, it is also important to avoid inadvertently reinforcing it. For example, if the child is fearful of dogs, it would only reinforce his/her fear to avoid dogs, perhaps commenting to the child, "There is a dog, Brian. I know you are afraid of dogs, so we will walk the other way to get away from it." This strategy may be a tempting one, as the parent may want to calm the child, but in the long run, this type of response will likely only intensify the fear (Garber et al., 1992).

Treatment of Fears and Specific Phobias

Treatment of fears and phobias typically involves behavioral techniques such as desensitization, modeling, and contingency management, as well as cognitive techniques such as using positive self-talk. Although there is empirical support for the efficacy of these techniques with school-age children and adolescents, research on preschool- and kindergarten-age children is lacking. However, it is likely that these techniques could work with younger children, as long as the clinician ensures that explanations and procedures are adapted to the cognitive level of the young child.

SYSTEMATIC DESENSITIZATION

Systematic desensitization involves a gradual exposure to the feared stimulus, combined with a response that is considered to be incompatible with anxiety (e.g., relaxation). Children first identify different situations in which they may encounter the feared object and rate the level of fear associated with each of these situations. These items are organized into a "fear hierarchy" (in which fears are listed from least to most feared), and the child is then exposed to the feared stimuli while simultaneously using an anxiety-relieving technique, such as progressive relaxation. This exposure can occur either in vivo (in the real-life setting) or through an imagined experience. This technique is one of the most commonly used, as well as one of the most efficacious, interventions for fears and phobias in children (American Academy of Child and Adolescent Psychiatry, 1997a; Morris & Kratochwill, 1998; Ollendick & King, 1998).

An example of a phobia of spiders is used throughout this section to illustrate the use of this procedure. The following is a dialogue between a clinician and a child about spiders. Sarah was referred to the clinician after she began to have extreme reactions to spiders, such as running away, crying, and screaming. This fear was interfering with her functioning, because she refused to engage in certain activities (e.g., playing in the yard with friends) for fear she would encounter a spider.

CLINICIAN: So, Sarah, tell me about spiders.

SARAH: Spiders are scary . . . I hate them.

CLINICIAN: What about spiders makes them scary?

SARAH: They're brown and hairy and have big legs and they eat people.

CLINICIAN: Uh-huh, and what else?

SARAH: I saw a movie where a kid got stuck in a web, and the spider bit him and ate him.

CLINICIAN: And what do you do when you see a spider?

SARAH: I run away and scream. One time I saw one at my preschool, and I hid in the bathroom.

Allowing the child to talk freely about what makes the stimulus scary for him/her and what he/she does when exposed to it is helpful in gathering more specific details about the child's phobia. Often, though, young children have difficulty elaborating on their phobias and their associated behaviors. Typically, the child's parents need to assist with the identification of the child's reactions to the feared object as well as the construction of the hierarchy. The fear hierarchy should begin with an item that produces little fear in the child (e.g., looking at a picture of a spider in a book) and end with the item that produces the most fear (e.g., touching a spider). The number of items included on the hierarchy are dependent upon the complexity of the child's fear.

Each of the items on the fear hierarchy should be rated by the child to determine the associated level of fear. For young children, it is often helpful to use a visual rating system, such as the one depicted in Figure 4.1., while asking the child "how full of fear" he or she is. The child might say that he/she is "full up to my knees" to indicate some fear, "full up to my stomach" to indicate a moderate amount of fear, or "full up to my head" to indicate more severe fear (Garber et al, 1992). It can be helpful to ask children a series of questions about their fear to understand under what circumstances they feel the most fearful. The following is an example of this kind of questioning, continuing with the conversation between the clinician and Sarah.

CLINICIAN: Sarah, I think I understand how scary spiders are for you. Using our system for how to rate your fear, how scary would you say you feel with us just talking about spiders?

SARAH: Up to my knees.

CLINICIAN: OK, and how about when you see a picture of a spider in a book?

SARAH: Up to my stomach. (*Points to her stomach.*)

CLINICIAN: OK, and how scary is it to see a TV show about spiders?

SARAH: Up to my shoulders.

CLINICIAN: I see. And how about when you actually see a spider on the wall?

SARAH: All the way up my neck. (*Points to her chin.*)

CLINICIAN: And to hold a spider?

SARAH: Past my head! (*Points to the ceiling.*)

Using this type of questioning, the clinician is able to develop a hierarchy of stimuli to work on with Sarah, such as the example provided in Table 4.1. It is important to note that creating such a list may make the child anxious and typically takes place over several sessions. As noted above, parents of young children typically are involved in the creation of the hierarchy. Parents can be asked to identify what objects/situations their child avoids on a regular basis and what stimuli lead to anxiety reactions (e.g., crying, clinging).

Once the hierarchy has been constructed, the clinician can begin to pair its items with a response that is incompatible with fear. Typically relaxation is used as this incompatible response. Following are summaries of relaxation techniques commonly used with children:

Deep Breathing. Stress tends to affect the bodies of adults and children alike in many ways. For example, people tend to take shorter, more shallow inhalations when anxious, in addition to taking fewer breaths ("forgetting to breathe"). A technique helpful to adults and

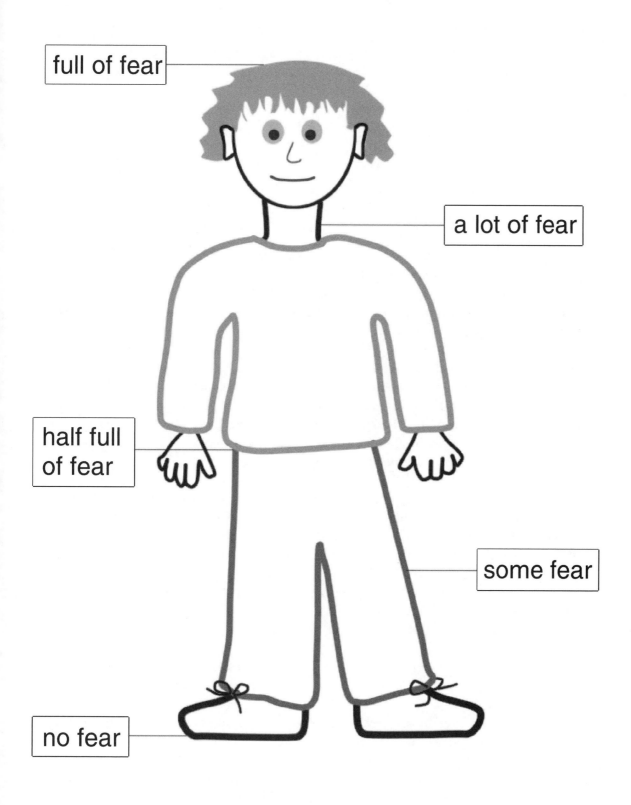

full of fear

a lot of fear

half full of fear

some fear

no fear

FIGURE 4.1. Visual aid for children self-assessing their current anxiety level. From Gretchen A. Gimpel and Melissa L. Holland (2003). Copyright by The Guilford Press. Permission to photocopy this figure is granted to purchasers of this book for personal use only (see copyright page for details).

TABLE 4.1. Hierarchy of Fears

Most fearful

Seeing a spider on the table next to me
Seeing a spider on the wall
Seeing a spider in a movie
Seeing a picture of a spider in a book
Saying the word spider

Least fearful

children is learning the art of deep breathing. To practice deep breathing with a child client, pick a quiet, private place to start. Both you and the child should lie on your backs. Have the child put one hand on his/her stomach, and one hand on the chest. When breathing correctly, the hand on the stomach should move up and down, but the hand on the chest does not. Model for the child the correct way to breath, instructing him/her to "fill up your stomach with air, like a balloon." Feedback is often necessary (e.g., "Do not arch your back or push out your stomach."). Let the child know that it can take a lot of practice to "belly breathe," and encourage the child to practice the skill every day and instruct the parents to praise the child when he/she does so. Once the skill has been mastered lying down, have the child practice the skill sitting down and standing up, as well as in different situations and contexts (Garber et al., 1992).

Slow Breathing. Once deep breathing has been mastered, the next step is to help the child slow down his/her breathing. A common technique is to count to four as the child breathes in, have the child hold his/her breath for four counts, breathe out for four counts, then hold the exhalation for four counts. Again, model for and practice with the child to aid him/her in the acquisition of the skill. A variation of this technique, particularly helpful if the child is struggling to understand the idea of slow breathing, is to have the child practice blowing bubbles. Typically, the slower the breath the more bubbles the child is able to produce.

Progressive Muscle Relaxation. When people are "stressed" or anxious, their muscles often tighten, leading to many physical complaints, such as headaches, backaches, leg aches, and stomachaches. Children tend to have many somatic, or physical, complaints when upset. Progressive muscle relaxation is one technique designed to relieve these physical symptoms—which, in turn, reduces the feelings of anxiety.

The first step of progressive muscle relaxation is to have the child sit comfortably or recline slightly in a comfortable chair. Practice the techniques of deep and slow breathing with the child to aid in initial relaxation. Let the child know that you will be doing a variety of different exercises to help relax muscles. It is preferable that the clinician do the exercises along with the child, modeling the correct postures and discussing the benefits of each pose. To add to the ease of implementing these techniques, a sample script is often used (see Figure 4.2). This script should be adapted, as needed, to fit the age and developmental level of each child. Slow, deep breathing should be used in between each exercise.

RELAXATION SCRIPT FOR YOUNG CHILDREN

Begin with breathing exercises.

Feet: Great job on your breathing. Now we are going to curl up our toes into tight little balls, just like this. They are like roly-polyies (potato bugs) curled up! Good. And hold it, and hold it [8–10 seconds]. Now release. Feel how warm and tingly your toes and feet feel. They are very relaxed now.

Legs: Now we are going to point our toes up and back toward our shins, like this. Feel how tight the backs of your legs feel? Kitty cats do this when they have just gotten up from a nap to stretch. Good, and hold it [8–10 seconds], and relax. Your legs feel so warm and good now.

Thighs: Now we are going to press our knees together and hold them really tight so that our legs feel really tight. Good, and press them harder, and hold it, and hold it [8–10 seconds], and release. Feel that warm, relaxed feeling now going down our legs and into our feet and toes.

Stomach: OK, now we are going to tighten our tummies really hard, like an elephant was going to step on our tummy, so we need it to be really tight, and hold it [8–10 seconds], and release. Feel how nice and comfortable that is?

Hands: Good, now we are going to curl our hands up into two tight balls by making tight fists, just like how roly-polys (potato bugs) roll up into tight little balls. And hold it, and make them tighter [8–10 seconds], and release. Feel that warm, tingly feeling in your fingers and hands?

Arms/Chest: Now we are going to put our hands together and press the palms of our hands into one another (model a praying position, with the hands over mid-chest). And press harder, and hold it [8–10 seconds], and release.

Shoulders: Let's put our shoulders up like we are trying to touch our shoulders to our ears. We look like monkeys when we do this! And hold them up, and up [8–10 seconds], and release. Feel that warm, relaxed feeling go down your shoulders, into your arms and hands, down through your stomach, and out your legs and toes. How warm and relaxed and calm our bodies feel.

Face: Now we will scrunch up our faces . . . tighten all of the muscles of your face—the cheeks, mouth, and nose muscles, the muscles of your forehead. How funny of a scrunched-up face can you make? Good! And hold it like that, hold it [8–10 seconds], and let go. Feel how good that feels.

End with breathing exercises.

FIGURE 4.2. Relaxation script for young children. From Gretchen A. Gimpel and Melissa L. Holland (2003). Copyright by The Guilford Press. Permission to photocopy this figure is granted to purchasers of this book for personal use only (see copyright page for details).

Imagery and fantasy may also be incorporated into a systematic desensitization protocol, as described below:

Imagery. After the deep breathing and/or progressive muscle relaxation, the use of imagery can be employed. Have the child imagine him/herself engaged in an activity that is fun and relaxing. If the child cannot think of any, suggest the image of the child swinging on a swing or playing at a playground or at the beach. Touch, scent, and sounds can be introduced in addition to the visual imagery of the child engaged in a pleasurable activity. For example, for the child imagining him/herself swinging, suggest how the child might feel the wind in his/her hair, hear the sounds of the playground, smell the sweet grass, and feel the tickle he/she may feel in the stomach when swinging really high.

Emotive Imagery. This technique involves identifying one of the child's superheroes and then incorporating this hero into a fantasy story involving the child. This story is then used instead of relaxation techniques, as the clinician works through the fear hierarchy.

Although relaxation and/or imagery are the most common "incompatible responses" used in systematic desensitization, it may not be feasible to use relaxation techniques with many preschool children, given their cognitive limitations. Alternatives to using relaxation techniques with younger children include playing with favorite toys, interacting with a favorite person, eating, or laughing (Schroeder & Gordon, 2002).

Once the child has practiced and mastered relaxation (or an alternative incompatible response has been chosen), the clinician can begin the next step of systematic desensitization by pairing the items on the fear hierarchy with the relaxation (or other similar) response. Have the child start with the first item on the hierarchy. Using our example of Sarah, she would say the word *spider* (see Table 4.1). Before and after she says the word, practice the relaxation skills with her, being sure to focus on the skills that provide her with the most relaxation. The premise behind this pairing is that a child cannot be anxious and relaxed at the same time (i.e., it is physiologically impossible). Therefore, having the child confront his/her phobias or fears while relaxed will disinhibit, or "turn off," the anxious response and make him/her feel more in control and less fearful of those objects or situations. This process typically takes time and often has to occur over the span of multiple sessions. Do not rush the process; allow ample time for the child to feel masterful over the first few items on the list before proceeding to the more feared items. The example below highlights the integration of these skills.

CLINICIAN: OK, Sarah, you did a great job of belly breathing and relaxing your muscles. You said that your fear feelings are at your "feet" right now, using our system of rating fear. Now I want you to say the word *spider*. Take in a deep breath, and as you exhale, say the word *spider*, like this. (*Does the exercise.*)

SARAH: (*Takes in a deep breath.*) *Spider.*

CLINICIAN: Good. Now take in a few more deep breaths and let them out. (*Models the deep breathing.*) Now I want you to tell me how much fear you have using our system. Is it at your feet, your knees, your stomach, your shoulders, your neck, or your head?

SARAH: My knees.

CLINICIAN: OK, let's take in a few more deep breaths and relax some muscles (*Proceeds to engage in some of the progressive muscle relaxation exercises.*) Now how would you rate your fear feelings?

SARAH: My feet.

CLINICIAN: OK, good. Let's have you take in another deep breath and let it out. Now, I want you to take in one more deep breath, but this time I want you to say the word *spider* while you breathe out, like this. (*Models.*)

SARAH: (*Takes in a deep breath.*) *Spider.*

CLINICIAN: Good, now let's do another deep breath and let it out. Now where would you rate your fear feelings?

SARAH: My feet.

CLINICIAN: Good, Sarah. Let's have you take in another deep breath, and as you let it out, again say *spider.*

As can be seen in this example, the clinician does not automatically proceed up the hierarchy but instead continues to focus on one area, until Sarah feels comfortable with it. Following this mastery, the clinician would introduce the next item on her hierarchy, "Seeing a picture of a spider in a book," and combine such a picture with the same relaxation techniques. Each session, the clinician would start with the beginning items on the hierarchy and work up, so that the child is not flooded at the beginning of the session. Praise and positive reinforcement should be given for any progress made.

As mentioned above, exposure can be either in vivo (graduated real-life exposure to the feared stimulus) or imaginal (having the child imagine the feared stimulus). Although in vivo exposure has some practical limitations, it has been found to be more efficacious in reducing phobic reactions for children than imaginal exposure. Results of studies examining in vivo exposure as compared to imaginal exposure found that for children ages 3–10, in vivo exposure was more effective than no-treatment or imaginal exposure modalities (Ollendick & King, 1998). In our example, Sarah would likely benefit more from gradual exposure to her feared stimulus (spiders) through books, photographs, plastic spiders, and real spiders, coupled with relaxation exercises, than if she imagined the items.

It is important that parents are involved in the treatment process with young children. (See Figure 4.3 for a parent handout on anxiety interventions.) Parents should be taught the incompatible response chosen so that they can help their child implement the technique at home when the child is faced with anxiety-provoking stimuli. Although parents can assist with exposure exercises, they should be instructed to avoid "rushing" the hierarchy. Parents should work with the child on what has been covered in therapy sessions. For example, a child with a dog phobia who has mastered looking at a picture of a dog in session should be allowed to practice this skill at home by looking at dog books and receiving praise for this accomplishment from his/her parents.

PARENT HANDOUT: TREATMENT OF ANXIETY

Many young children have fears. Typical fears exhibited by preschool-and kindergarten-age children include fear of the dark, fear of specific animals, and fear of separation from parents (or other caregivers). Fears are not unusual in young children, but when a fear begins to interfere with the child's functioning (e.g., the child refuses to attend school) or the family's functioning (e.g., parents argue about how to address a fear), then treatment should be considered. Below are some common intervention techniques for fears and ways you, as a parent, can assist with treatment. Make sure first to discuss your use of these techniques with your child's clinician.

Systematic Desensitization

This technique involves gradually exposing your child to a feared object, while having your child engage in an activity that is incompatible with fear. Relaxation is used as the incompatible response with older children. Relaxation may be used with young children, but other fun activities, such as blowing bubbles, running around the yard, or playing a short game also can be used.

It is important not to rush the exposure exercises but to start with exposure to situations in which the child is unlikely to exhibit a high level of fear. For example, for a child with a fear of dogs, the child might first look at pictures of a dog, then observe a dog outside, then be in the same room as a dog, then touch the dog.

Your child's clinician will help you set up a systematic desensitization program. The clinician may work with your child on exposure exercises during session and also may have you conduct some exposure exercises at home.

Positive Self-Talk

Pay attention to what your child says and help him/her replace negative thoughts with more positive ones. For example, if your child says, "I can't go outside because there might be a dog and dogs are scary," you can respond with, "Dogs can be scary, but the dogs outside are nice and you're brave. Tell yourself that you're brave, and that you'll be okay outside." When using this approach, make sure you do not minimize or belittle your child's fear. The goal is to acknowledge the fear while putting a more positive "spin" on the child's thoughts.

Modeling

Make sure to model appropriate (nonfearful) interactions for your child. If your child is afraid of dogs and the friendly neighbor dog comes along while you are outside with your child, talk out loud to the dog, saying such things as "You're a nice, friendly dog—I'd like to pet you."

Contingency Management

Using this approach, you would reinforce your child for gradually interacting with the feared object. For example, if your child is afraid of dogs, you might initially reinforce your child for looking out the window at the neighbor's dog, then standing in the yard with the dog for a brief period of time, then standing in the yard for a longer period of time, etc. You can use stickers or candy as reinforcers, but also make sure to provide your child with verbal praise (e.g., "Great job hanging out in the yard with Rufus. You're so brave.")

FIGURE 4.3. Parent handout: Treatment of Anxiety. From Gretchen A. Gimpel and Melissa L. Holland (2003). Copyright by The Guilford Press. Permission to photocopy this figure is granted to purchasers of this book for personal use only (see copyright page for details).

OTHER INTERVENTION TECHNIQUES FOR FEARS AND PHOBIAS

As noted previously, although systematic desensitization is the most commonly used technique for fears and phobias, other techniques have also been found to be effective. Because of the potential difficulties with using systematic desensitization with young children, some of these other techniques (reviewed below), or a combination of techniques may be warranted.

Positive Self-Talk. Using positive self-statements can be an excellent tool for the anxious (or depressed) child to help him/her feel more positive and self-assured in a variety of situations. Make a list of positive statements the child can make about him/herself or the situation. For each negative thought or statement, a positive thought should be developed. For example, for the child afraid to go to preschool, the child could say to him/herself, "I am not afraid," "I will be OK until my daddy picks me up," or "I am brave and will make friends." It is important to have the child practice the positive self-talk often. Have the child begin by saying the statements out loud, then try to switch the child to internal self-talk before he/she goes into the social situation (e.g., saying the statements in his/her head or softly to him/herself).

Modeling. Modeling is a well-researched and frequently used technique that allows the child to observe an individual interacting with the feared stimulus in a nonfearful manner. For example, a child with a dog phobia may watch another child pet a dog. Modeling can either be live or symbolic. In live modeling, the child observes an actual person interacting with the feared stimulus. In symbolic modeling, the model is either presented on video or the child imagines the model. Participant modeling, in which the child engages in the behavior with the model (e.g., the child also begins to pet the dog) also can be used. Often other techniques, such as positive self-talk and deep breathing, are used along with modeling (Knell, 2000; Ollendick & King, 1998). For example, in participant modeling, the model may begin to approach the dog, saying, "I'm feeling kind of scared, but it's going to be okay. I know I can get a little closer to the dog." Following this, the child would be encouraged to approach the dog, using similar coping/positive self-talk statements.

Research with children ages 3–5 years has shown that children in a group format, in which models approached the feared stimulus while the fearful children watched, had significantly less fear and more approach behaviors to the stimulus than children who were exposed to the feared stimulus without a model. Both filmed modeling and live modeling have been found to be efficacious procedures for treating excessive fears and phobias. Participant modeling has been shown to be even more effective than either symbolic or live modeling without a guided participation component (Ollendick & King, 1998). Although same-age peers are typically used as models, parents, teachers, and other adults also can serve as models by allowing the child to observe them coping in a nonfearful way with the feared stimulus.

Contingency Management. Contingency management is another commonly used technique for working with children who display phobic behaviors. Shaping and positive reinforcement are the most commonly used contingency management techniques to reduce phobic behaviors in young children (Ollendick & King, 1998). Shaping involves reinforcing successive approximations toward the target behavior. For example, in the case of the child who has a phobia of dogs, the child would be reinforced first for being in the same room with the dog, then reinforced for approaching the dog, and finally reinforced for petting the dog. Positive reinforcement, such as praise and/or tangible reinforcers (e.g., small toys or stickers), would be used to strengthen and maintain any gains made. Charts can be helpful in visually demonstrating the child's accomplishments in combating the fear. For example, for the child with the dog phobia, a winding road could be drawn on a piece of poster board, with different accomplishments noted along the road (e.g., looking at a dog in a book, being in the room with a dog, approaching the dog, petting the dog) and a small marker moved along the road as the child accomplishes these steps.

In a review of the research on the use of contingency management techniques, Ollendick and King (1998) concluded that reinforced practice (gradual exposure with reinforcement) was shown to be more effective than no-treatment and superior to live modeling and verbal coping skills treatment modalities. Contingency management methods may be particularly useful with preschool- and kindergarten-age children who may have difficulties with some of the other techniques (e.g., positive-self talk, relaxation techniques) that have more of a cognitive component.

Separation Anxiety, Including Early School or Daycare Refusal

At one time or another, almost all children experience some form of anxiety when separated from primary caregivers. In fact, this separation anxiety is developmentally appropriate during the toddler years (18–24 months). Toddlers often cry, cling, and have temper tantrums when they are about to be separated from their parents. Some children, however, will continue to have these anxiety symptoms beyond this developmental stage (Paige, 1998). As mentioned previously in this chapter, the essential feature of separation anxiety is an excessive anxiety concerning separation from the home or from those to whom the child is attached, beyond that expected for the child's developmental level, and lasting for a period of at least 4 weeks (American Psychiatric Association, 1994).

The initial separation that occurs when children begin daycare or school can be stressful for all children. The unfamiliar surroundings and people, along with the separation from their parents, results in initial feelings of uneasiness for many children. Most children overcome their feelings of anxiety and quickly begin to enjoy their new setting. For those children who continue to exhibit symptoms of separation anxiety at the time of separation or in anticipation of separation, intervention is imperative. The following sections outline how to prevent and treat such problems. Although the interventions described in this section are contextualized for the school or daycare setting, many of these techniques also can be used when a child displays anxiety about being left with a babysitter or unfamiliar relative or when entering any new situation about which the child is fearful.

Prevention of Separation Anxiety

Before their child enters a new setting, parents can take steps to help prevent any significant anxieties from forming. Obviously the parents must first feel comfortable with the upcoming situation. Parents should carefully select the daycare or preschool setting their child is to attend, ideally visiting several different settings to evaluate which type of setting is best for both the parent and the child. Interviewing the daycare providers/teachers and observing a "typical" day in the new setting can give parents a feeling of security and comfort, which in turn helps the child to begin to feel confident. If the child is anxious about having a new babysitter, it is often a good idea for the babysitter to visit with the child while the parents are in the home to help familiarize the child with the new person. Likewise, parents should consider taking their child to a new daycare or school setting in advance to familiarize the child with the new surroundings. A weekend or evening trip can be helpful to see the building and the yard area and help ease the child into the new setting.

It is important for parents to convey a genuinely positive attitude about the new setting or situation to their child. Discussing some of the exciting things that take place in that environment (such as games, art projects, and field trips) with their child can be helpful. The teacher's, babysitter's or daycare provider's name should be used in these conversations to familiarize the child with the new adult.

On the "big day," the parent should accompany the child to the new setting and stay with the child for a short while so that he/she does not feel abandoned. If the parent is having difficulties letting go, arrange to have another adult with whom the child is familiar accompany him/her. Encourage the child to engage in the initial activities of the day. If the child shows no difficulty joining in, the parent should let the child know that he/she will return to pick up the child at the end of the day. The parent should make certain that he/she is *not late* picking up the child, particularly during the first several days.

After the day at daycare, school, or with the new sitter, the parent should allow some time for the child to discuss his/her day in the new setting or situation, responding with enthusiasm to the information the child shares. Praise the child for his/her accomplishments and place any materials and art projects the child has brought home on the refrigerator door or in a scrap book to "show off" the child's achievements.

Treatment of Separation Anxiety

The first indication of a separation anxiety disorder, as related to daycare or school, is often refusal to go to school. The child may state this refusal directly by indicating that he/she does not want to go to the new setting any longer and that he/she would prefer to stay home with the parent. Often, though, the child's anxiety may be communicated in a more indirect manner. The child may complain of stomachaches or headaches in the morning or throw temper tantrums when the parent is getting the child ready for daycare/ preschool. Typically the child also becomes quite clingy when the parent attempts to leave the child at daycare/preschool.

If the child does voice specific concerns about the daycare/preschool setting, it is important for the adult to listen carefully and determine their validity. If a child notes, for example, that his/her daycare provider is "mean," it would be important to ask the child to describe *mean*. For instance, the parent could say to the child, "Sophia, it sounds like you feel Ms. Thompson is mean. What does she do that is mean?" This can aid the adult in ruling out any maltreatment that is occurring in the setting. If necessary, the parent could make unannounced visits to the setting to observe how the adults interact with the children and to determine if anything seems unusual about the setting. Though rare, maltreatment can occur in daycare and school settings and, if suspected, it is essential to investigate further and, if necessary, place the child in a different setting. Most often, though, the child is simply having anxiety about the setting, and this anxiety must be addressed before it becomes more serious.

It is important to note that not all cases of school refusal are due to separation anxiety. If the child's worry is centered on something specific occurring in the daycare, such as teasing from other children (as opposed to anxiety about separating from the parent), this child may be exhibiting a school phobia. Children with a school phobia usually have fears associated with a specific concern, whereas with separation anxiety, the worries are focused primarily on separation from the parent. If the child is able to pinpoint a specific concern, the parent should address the concern with the daycare provider or teacher as soon as possible (Paige, 1998).

The physical complaints that are typical in young children may initially be mistaken for real physical problems. Though obviously many children do catch colds and other illnesses, it is important for parents to determine, as soon as possible, if the child is feigning illness. Clues parents can look for include (but are not limited to): frequent morning sickness before school or daycare, then miraculously "getting better" once he/she is allowed to stay home; no physical signs of illness, such as a runny nose or fever; frequent complaints of illness during the weekdays or before returning to the avoided setting, but no illness reported during days spent with the parent; and empathetic pleas from the child that he/she feels ill just before returning to the daycare or school setting, when previously the child seemed fine. A visit to the pediatrician to rule out any medical illness also is an appropriate step a parent can take. If there is no medical reason the child should be absent, the child should be returned to the daycare or school setting.

It is extremely important that parents and other adults do not reinforce the child's anxious and avoidant behaviors. The child should be reinforced for attending school via positive reinforcement (e.g., praise), and parents should ignore behaviors the child engages in to attempt to get out of going to school (e.g., crying, whining). In addition, parents may want to set up a system in which the child can earn tangible reinforcers for going to school without exhibiting negative behaviors. (See Figure 4.4 for a parent handout detailing the treatment of separation anxiety disorder.)

In the following steps, a case example of Tim, who was refusing to attend kindergarten, is used to illustrate the treatment for separation anxiety.

PARENT HANDOUT: SEPARATION ANXIETY AND SCHOOL REFUSAL

Young children often have difficulty separating from their parents. When separation is anticipated, they may engage in behaviors such as clinginess, crying, and throwing tantrums. Refusal to go to school is frequently seen as part of separation anxiety disorder. However, school refusal also can be due to other problems, such as fear of the school or a specific individual at the school. In children with separation anxiety disorder, fear of separating from the caregiver is the main anxiety, and this is expressed in any situation in which separation is anticipated (e.g., at school, with a babysitter). Although some anxiety is typical when children are first introduced to a new situation (e.g., when they begin school), it is important to intervene if these symptoms do not go away.

Prevention of Separation Anxiety

To help prevent distress upon separation and to decrease the chances that separation anxiety will develop, the following steps can be taken when your child is introduced to a new situation, such as daycare or preschool:

1. Select a daycare or preschool with which you are comfortable and familiar.
2. Discuss with your child positive activities that will take place in the new setting (e.g., playing games, meeting new people).
3. Accompany your child to the new setting and stay with him/her for a *short* period of time.
4. After you pick up your child, praise him/her for doing well in school and allow your child a chance to talk about what happened during the day.

Treatment of Separation Anxiety/School Refusal

Children with separation anxiety typically engage in behaviors to attempt to prevent separation from occurring. The child may directly state his/her refusal to attend school, but more frequently this refusal is communicated through indirect methods such as complaints of stomachaches or headaches in the morning or throwing temper tantrums when you are getting the child ready for daycare/preschool. Typically the child also becomes quite clingy when you attempt to leave him/her at daycare/preschool. If your child is exhibiting such behaviors, it is important to address the problem immediately.

1. Do not reinforce the child's anxious and avoidant behaviors. *This is very important.* Do not allow your child to stay home from school unless he/she truly is sick. Do not give in to whining and crying and allow your child to stay home.
2. If you have been allowing your child to stay home, immediately return your child to school and do not allow him/her to miss future days of school.
3. Give your child a "transitional object" to help him/her get through the day. A transitional object is an item given by a parent to remind the child of the parent. Some examples of objects include a locket with a photograph of the parent in it, a "lucky penny," a "power ring," or a note or picture drawn by the parent to help the child feel special, loved, and powerful.
4. Forewarn the daycare provider or teacher about your child's separation anxiety.
5. Reinforce your child for having attended daycare/school.

Consistency is key to resolving your child's school refusal behavior. If you have allowed your child to stay out of school for a long time or if your child has severe anxiety symptoms, a more gradual exposure to the school setting may be necessary. For example, you might first have your child go to school for an hour each day and gradually work up to having him/her there for the whole school day. However, in most cases immediate and full return to the school setting is best.

FIGURE 4.4. Parent handout: Separation Anxiety and School Refusal. From Gretchen A. Gimpel and Melissa L. Holland (2003). Copyright by The Guilford Press. Permission to photocopy this figure is granted to purchasers of this book for personal use only (see copyright page for details).

1. The night before Tim was to return to school, his parents told him that tomorrow he would be going back to school. His parents ignored Tim's cries, tantrums, and pleas to stay home.

2. The next morning, his parents got Tim up, helped him dress, fed him breakfast, and told him, in a matter-of-fact manner, that his mother would be dropping him off at the school on her way to work. Again, all pleas for not going to school by Tim were completely ignored.

3. Tim was given a "transitional object" to help him feel safe in the school setting. A transitional object is an item given by a primary attachment figure to remind the child of the caregiver. Examples include a locket with photograph of the parent in it, a "lucky penny," a "power ring," or a note or picture drawn by the parent to help the child feel special, loved, and powerful. Tim's father gave him a lucky penny to keep in his pocket to help him feel "strong" and "happy" throughout his day, until they could see each other again that night.

4. Tim's parents had forewarned his teacher about his separation anxiety, and she helped to comfort Tim that day. Though Tim cried frequently that day and isolated himself from others, he was able to stay in the classroom for the whole day. When he played a game with the other children, she praised him.

5. Tim's mother picked Tim up after his school day and spoke with the teacher about how he had managed. Both parents reinforced Tim that evening for his day at school. They told him that they knew it was hard for him to have gone, but that each day it would get easier. With effort, Tim's parents were able to ignore the tantrums and pleas Tim engaged in that evening about not wanting to attend school again.

6. The next morning Tim launched into the same behaviors of screaming, crying, and refusing to go to school. Tim's parents continued with the routine they had implemented the day before, and, once again, dropped Tim off at school. Upon picking Tim up from school, his teacher told his mother that Tim had been able to join the rest of the children more that day than the previous day. Tim's mother and father reinforced this accomplishment by taking Tim out to his favorite restaurant that night.

7. It took several weeks of this routine before Tim began to attend school without argument and with a positive attitude. Tim had conquered his separation anxiety and was able to have a positive Kindergarten experience.

As seen in this case example, parental consistency was key to Tim's returning to the school setting. For children whose parents have allowed them to stay out of school for a long time because of the anxiety symptoms or for children with severe anxiety symptoms, a more gradual exposure to the school setting may be necessary. For example, the child might first go to school for an hour each day and gradually work up to staying for the whole school day. However, in most cases immediate and full return to school is appropriate. Returning the child to the avoided setting is the primary intervention used in the treatment of separation anxiety disorder (American Academy of Child and Adolescent Psychiatry, 1997a). Other techniques that may be used in addition to this include:

Technique	Examples
Relaxation techniques	Deep and slow breathing techniques Progressive muscle relaxation Guided imagery
Positive self-talk	"I can do it." "I am not afraid."
Sticker charts	Sticker for each school day attended; once a certain number of stickers is obtained, the child earns a special reinforcer (e.g., going to McDonald's after school with Mom)
Contracts	A written agreement that if the child attends school without throwing a tantrum in the morning, he/she can watch an hour of TV after school

Selective Mutism

Children with selective mutism fail to speak in specific settings, such as school or daycare, but they speak in other settings, such as their home. This disturbance must have lasted for at least 1 month, is not limited to the first month of school, and the failure to speak is not due to a lack of knowledge or comfort with the spoken language required in the social situation (American Psychiatric Association, 1994). Other behaviors, such as excessive shyness, social isolation and withdrawal, negativism, anxiety, oppositional defiant behaviors, and throwing tantrums also may be present (Kehle & Bray, 1998). The onset of the selective mutism typically occurs before the age of 5 and is commonly first recognized when the child enters the preschool or kindergarten setting. Although selective mutism is not classified as an anxiety disorder, it is often considered to have an anxiety component.

If the child appears to be losing language capabilities across settings, or if the child appears to be distressed about the loss of language or the difficulties in speaking, it is important that he/she be evaluated as soon as possible by a physician to rule out any neurological impairment. If the lack of speech appears to be related to unfamiliarity with the English language, then the child should be referred to an appropriate alternative language program. If the failure to speak appears to be directly related to a language problem (e.g., stuttering or another communication disorder), then the child should be referred to a speech and language specialist. When attempting to determine whether the lack of speech is due to selective mutism or one of these other possible causes, the fact that normal speech occurs in some settings is the key indicator of selective mutism.

Causes and Prevention of Selective Mutism

Explanations for the causes of selective mutism vary, though it is likely that the child has been reinforced for his/her silence via negative reinforcement (i.e., the child is allowed to escape or avoid an aversive task by not talking), thereby making the behavior highly resistant to intervention. For example, peers in the child's class may begin to "interpret" the mute child's needs to others, the child may receive special attention (i.e., positive reinforcement) for not speaking, and the teacher may withhold making requests of the child if the requests seem to upset or bother him/her (Kehle & Bray, 1998). Thus, to help prevent selective mutism, adults should require that the child answers on his/her own; if the child does not, adults should ensure that he/she is not receiving special attention or being allowed to escape a task because of the lack of talking. Often, though, selective mutism is not fully recognized until it has become a significant problem.

Treatment of Selective Mutism

The school setting is the most common one in which children exhibit selective mutism. Obviously a child who does not speak at school poses a significant educational problem, and treatment should be implemented promptly. The most effective treatments for selective mutism are behaviorally based interventions implemented in the school environment. Hence, school psychologists are likely to be the targeted professional for educating parents and teachers about the disorder and designing the intervention strategies.

The most common treatment for selective mutism is the shaping and generalization of speaking behaviors. *Shaping* refers to the positive reinforcement of successive approximations to the target behavior—in this case, audible speech. Positive reinforcement strategies may include verbal praise, attention given to the child, a sticker, small toy, or other reward. The successive approximations that may be reinforced include the child responding to a question (1) with one-word answers, (2) with several-word answers, and (3) by spontaneously offering an answer. For example, at the initial stages of treatment, the teacher may ask the child "What color crayon would you like to draw with?" then provide the crayon and verbal praise when the child answers "Red." Later the child may be asked more complex questions that require more wordy responses.

In addition to requiring limited speech initially, intervention programs also may involve select peers at the beginning stages of treatment. For example, instead of being expected to speak in front of the whole classroom, the child may initially be prompted to speak in small group activities. Once the child begins to speak in a small group, more children are gradually added to the group.

As described previously, it is important to eliminate any reinforcement the child receives for not speaking. The child should not be allowed to point or make other signals for things he/she wants; indeed *all* nonverbal attempts to communicate should be ignored. Other students in the class should not be allowed to "speak for" the child; instead, the child's peers should be told that the child must now speak for him/herself.

As the child begins to speak more frequently and in the presence of more people, the prompts and reinforcers that were previously used are gradually "faded out." It is important to continue with the reinforcement of verbal behaviors and the consistent ignoring of noncommunicative behaviors until the child demonstrates verbal fluency and appears to find spoken language reinforcing, in and of itself (e.g., others respond to the child's verbal requests; the child appears to be making friends; the teacher positively responds to the child's answering of a question).

Another strategy that can be used as a supplement involves having the child invite a school friend to his/her house over the weekend,with the parents reinforcing verbal communication or play between the two of them. It is hoped that the child will then begin to be verbal with this peer in the school setting as well. If the child is verbal with his/her siblings, the teacher can invite the siblings into the classroom after school and allow the child and the siblings to play a game. Assuming the previously mute child becomes verbal during the game, the teacher can then begin to include some of the child's classmates in the game (Kehle & Bray, 1998).

At times the child's parents are not aware of the full extent of their child's difficulties in the school setting, because the child converses freely at home. Volunteering in the child's classroom can help parents see the extent and pervasiveness of the child's problem and form a collaborative connection with the school personnel. Parents should only reinforce verbal behaviors and encourage their child to speak for him/herself in different settings (Garber et al., 1992).

Though often successful, these techniques take time and considerable energy on the part of the teacher, other students, parents, and professionals working with the child. It is extremely important that, once in place, the intervention techniques continue until the child's selective mutism has resolved. Inconsistency likely will only strengthen the child's mutism.

OVERVIEW OF DEPRESSIVE SYMPTOMS

Feeling sad or depressed at times is a normal occurrence for both children and adults. Occasional depressed mood can occur at any age and can have a variety of causes. Most young children who experience a depressed mood recover quickly, with the sadness lasting for only a brief period of time. No intervention is likely warranted for these children. However, some children have a more pervasive depressed mood that does not remit and interferes with daily living activities, including interpersonal relationships and decreased school and home functioning. The prevalence of severe depression in children is about 5–6%, though exact figures, particularly for younger children, are not known (Saklofske, Janzen, Hildebrand, & Kaufmann, 1998). Younger children tend to have lower prevalence rates of depression than do older children; rates for preadolescent children are estimated to be less than 3%. However, because preschoolers are rarely included in prevalence studies of depression, the rates of the disorder in this population are unknown, although they are likely quite low (Hammen & Rudolph, 2003).

The DSM-IV states that the "core symptoms of a Major Depressive Episode are the same for children and adolescents, although there are data that suggest that the prominence of characteristic symptoms may change with age" (American Psychiatric Association, 1994, p. 324). Symptoms commonly seen in young children include irritability, social withdrawal, and somatic complaints. However, young children also can experience the core symptoms of depressed mood and loss of pleasure or interest in activities during the day. Other symptoms young children may exhibit include weight loss or gain (including a failure to make expected weight gains in young children), insomnia or hypersomnia, loss of energy, psychomotor agitation, and difficulties concentrating. The child must have had some of these symptoms for at least 2 weeks for the symptoms to be considered a depressive episode. A long-term mild depression (lasting at least 1 year for children) is called dysthymia, whereas a depressed mood that occurs in response to a specific stressor and resolves usually within 6 months is called an adjustment disorder with depressed mood (American Psychiatric Association, 1994).

Prevention of Childhood Depression

The prevention of chronic childhood depression begins with early recognition of the signs and symptoms of depression. Teachers, parents, daycare workers, and other adults in the child's life can all play an integral role in identifying when a child appears depressed. The young child typically has difficulty understanding or verbalizing his/her thoughts and feelings. It has been shown, however, that children as young as the age of 3 can accurately identify their emotions, and children by the age of 5 are able to verbalize their feelings instead of acting upon them (Luby, 2000).

Increasing the support to the child and paying attention to factors that could be contributing to the child's change in functioning are important. For example, if the child is being bullied by another student at school, the teacher should intervene in the classroom as well as alert the child's parents about what is happening. Signs and symptoms of child abuse, as discussed in Chapter 6, are also important factors to attend to, especially for teachers and daycare workers, and should be reported if suspected.

Treatment of Depressive Symptoms

The treatment for depression in adolescents and adults typically includes a variety of cognitive-behavioral techniques. Although these techniques have been used with children with some success, such techniques have not been investigated for use with preschool- and kindergarten-age children. Given the cognitive component of these techniques, it may be difficult to impossible to implement them with young children. Instead, a multifaceted approach, which includes parent education and family systems work, is often recommended (American Academy of Child and Adolescent Psychiatry, 1998).

Establishing an effective therapeutic alliance with the parents early on is important in maintaining the involvement of the family and child in treatment. A major component of fostering this alliance is to educate the parent on the disorder of childhood depression and its course and treatment. This form of education often leads to a discussion of issues that could be maintaining the child's depression, such as family problems or parental depression. Children who have a parent who is depressed may be more likely to exhibit depressive symptoms themselves (Kaslow, Morris, & Rehm, 1998). If parent psychopathology is an issue, individual treatment for the parent should be recommended in addition to treating the child's depressive symptoms. In addition, a poor parent–child relationship or general family dysfunction can contribute to a child's depressive symptoms (Kaslow et al., 1998).

The type of treatment used with the young child largely rests on what types of symptoms the child is exhibiting and what seems to be maintaining the depression. A careful assessment should be conducted by the clinician to determine what is happening for that child. The clinician also should determine how the young child is currently feeling via the use of pictures or feelings charts. An example of a feelings chart is provided in Figure 4.5. In addition, Figure 4.6 depicts a chart that may be used on a daily basis (with the parent assisting the child) to track the child's moods across time.

If the young child appears to have many negative thoughts and low self-esteem, these thoughts need to be challenged supportively and replaced by more positive thoughts (i.e., cognitive restructuring). Gentle questioning about different topics may reveal where the child's faulty thinking lies. Often the child is repeating to him/herself a negative statement told to him/her by a peer, sibling, or parent. The following example illustrates this technique of challenging and replacing negative faulty thinking. This example involves Ashley, a 5-year-old who has been saying that she is "stupid" while in session with her clinician.

ASHLEY: I can't do this puzzle. I'm stupid.

CLINICIAN: You think that you are stupid? What makes you think that?

ASHLEY: We had to do puzzles at school, and I couldn't do that puzzle either.

CLINICIAN: Yeah, some puzzles can be pretty tricky.

ASHLEY: All puzzles are tricky for me because I'm dumb.

CLINICIAN: I also know that different people are really good at different things, and not so good at other things. It does not mean that people are stupid, it just means that they might be better at something else.

ASHLEY: Yeah, but I'm not good at anything.

CLINICIAN: Didn't you just tell me that you learned to ride your bike over the weekend and that you were good at that? I also remember that clay dog you made in here last week and how good that was. You brought that in for show-and-tell yesterday, right?

ASHLEY: Yeah, everyone said it was really good.

CLINICIAN: So I guess you aren't stupid, you're just good at different things besides puzzles. If you ever think to yourself "I am stupid," you need to say to yourself , "I'm not stupid, I'm good at lots of things." Then tell yourself what you are good at doing. Let's practice saying that. I'm good at doing a lot of things like . . .

ASHLEY: I'm good at doing lots of things, like riding my bike.

CLINICIAN: Great job, Ashley.

If the child appears agitated and restless, deep breathing and other relaxation techniques can be useful for the young child to practice both in and out of session. Examples of these techniques were provided earlier in this chapter. Training the parents to model the use of these techniques for their child at home is another way to encourage the child to practice these techniques.

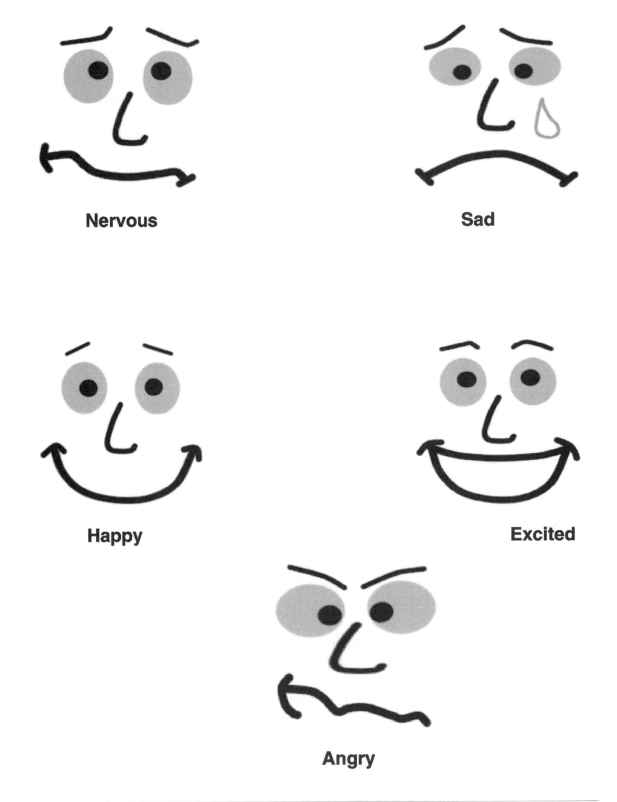

Nervous

Sad

Happy

Excited

Angry

FIGURE 4.5. Feelings chart for preschoolers and kindergarteners. From Gretchen A. Gimpel and Melissa L. Holland (2003). Copyright by The Guilford Press. Permission to photocopy this figure is granted to purchasers of this book for personal use only (see copyright page for details).

DAILY FEELINGS CHART

CIRCLE HOW YOU ARE FEELING

Monday					
	Nervous	Sad	Happy	Excited	Angry

Tuesday					
	Nervous	Sad	Happy	Excited	Angry

Wednesday					
	Nervous	Sad	Happy	Excited	Angry

Thursday					
	Nervous	Sad	Happy	Excited	Angry

Friday					
	Nervous	Sad	Happy	Excited	Angry

Saturday					
	Nervous	Sad	Happy	Excited	Angry

Sunday					
	Nervous	Sad	Happy	Excited	Angry

FIGURE 4.6. Daily feelings chart for preschoolers and kindergarteners. From Gretchen A. Gimpel and Melissa L. Holland (2003). Copyright by The Guilford Press. Permission to photocopy this figure is granted to purchasers of this book for personal use only (see copyright page for details).

Because of the young child's cognitive level, it may be difficult to implement techniques such as cognitive restructuring and relaxation training. However, some interventions actively involve parents and therefore may be more appropriate for preschool- and kindergarten-age children. Scheduling pleasurable activities is a frequently recommended intervention for depression whereby parents are instructed to ensure that their child is engaged in a number of active and fun endeavors. For example, parents can suggest that the child invite a friend from school or daycare over to the house for several hours on a weekend or after school. This strategy is particularly appropriate if the child is socially isolated in the home (e.g., no siblings around the child's age and no neighborhood peers). Involving the child in a new interest or craft—instead of watching TV—also can be useful, especially if a significant adult in the child's life can help out with, or participate in, the activity and can give positive reinforcement and praise to the child for engaging in the activity. Other activities parents may engage their child in include drawing, singing, dancing, playing with clay, simple board games, painting, riding a tricycle, or engaging in other outdoor physical activities. Anything that the child finds fun and enjoyable (or previously found to be so, if the child has demonstrated a decreased interest in activities as part of his/her depressive symptoms) should be encouraged.

Parents should provide a great deal of positive reinforcement while engaged in pleasurable activities with their child. Parents should also look for opportunities to praise and encourage other appropriate non-depressive behaviors. In addition, if the parent hears the child make a self-critical statement, the parent can gently and supportively challenge that statement (Saklofske et al., 1998). For families in which there is a poor parent–child relationship that may be contributing to the depression, setting up a structured positive play activity (such as that described in Chapter 3) may be beneficial for both the parent and the child. Because a lack of structure may contribute to depression in children, it is also important that the parent maintain a regular routine for the child, including mealtimes, bedtimes, and activity times. Minimizing changes within the family as much as possible and talking with the child about impending changes before they occur also may help to minimize the child's worry.

Teachers and daycare workers can assist in helping the depressed child in several ways: (1) allowing the child to sit next to friends or potential friends during rug time, lunch, or class time; (2) avoiding situations in which the child could be socially isolated (e.g., when students choose teams for group projects or games); (3) giving frequent praise and positive reinforcement in class; and (4) helping the child focus on the positives instead of the negatives (Saklofske et al., 1998). In addition, the teacher can model coping statements. For example, if the depressed child states, "I can never do anything right" as he/she crumbles up the art project, the teacher can state, "This project is tricky, and a lot of my students have had a hard time with it. Let's see if we can try and do it together." This approach allows the child to "save face"—after all, the project has been perceived as "tricky" by other students—while still providing an opportunity for the child to succeed in the project. Once the child has successfully completed the project, the teacher should lavish praise on him/her; when other similar projects come up, the teacher can remind the child of the great work he/she did on the last project.

CHAPTER SUMMARY

Although the treatment of internalizing disorders in young children has traditionally been overlooked by mental health professionals, more attention has been brought to this important area over the last few years. This chapter provided an overview of commonly used prevention methods and treatment modalities for use with preschool- and kindergarten-age children experiencing anxiety and depression. Although research on the use of these techniques specifically with young children is still needed, there is a growing body of literature attesting to the effectiveness of cognitive-behavioral techniques with school-age children. By simplifying the language used, involving parents and teachers in the treatment plan, and using concrete examples, these same techniques can be helpful for this young population.

5

Managing and Preventing
Everyday Problems

Some of the problems that cause the most stress and concern for parents of preschool- and kindergarten-age children are behaviors that relate to routines that are part of everyday life, such as eating, sleeping, and using the bathroom appropriately. Although problems in these areas are often transitory and may not be severe enough or atypical enough to warrant a formal diagnosis, providing treatment can alleviate significant parent and child stress and potentially lead to a more positive parent–child relationship. In addition, management of such problems while the child is young may prevent later adverse outcomes in those situations in which the problem is not transitory. In the sections below, treatment of these problems is outlined.

TOILETING

Toilet Training

Toilet training is an important developmental milestone for preschool-age children. For most children this task is accomplished with relatively little difficulty. However, many parents have questions and/or concerns regarding this process. Unfortunately, there is little scientific literature regarding how to toilet train or how to address problems associated with toilet training. One question parents commonly ask is when they should begin toilet training their child. Although there are no clear guidelines to follow, toilet training should not be initiated until the child is both physiologically and psychologically ready for it. In infancy the bladder empties as a reflex; the baby has no control over this action. In the toddler years, children begin to become aware of when their bladders are full. By age 3 most children are able to control their sphincter muscles voluntarily and inhibit urination during the day; nighttime control comes a year or 2 later. Children are typically considered to have achieved bladder control when they can remain dry for several hours, empty their bladders completely when urinating, and demonstrate some realization that they need to urinate (Howe & Walker, 1992; Kuhn, Marcus, & Pitner, 1999). For most children, toilet training occurs some time between the ages of 2 and 4.

In addition to physiological readiness, children must exhibit other aspects of readiness before toilet training can be successful. For example, children must be able to perform the motor movements required for toileting, such as walking to the bathroom, removing the appropriate clothing, and sitting on the toilet (Howe & Walker, 1992; Kuhn et al., 1999). They must have some basic language skills and be able to understand and communicate the words related to toileting. In addition, the ability to follow parental instructions is important to successful toilet training. Children who are noncompliant and exhibit disruptive behaviors will be difficult to toilet train. If a parent is having difficulty toilet training his/her child, behavioral characteristics of the child need to be assessed and, if necessary, parent training (see Chapter 3) implemented prior to toilet training, so that the child first learns to comply to parental commands (Kuhn et al., 1999).

There are two basic approaches to toilet training: the child-oriented approach advocated by Brazelton (1962), and the structured behavioral approach pioneered by Azrin and Foxx (1974). In the child-oriented approach, toilet training is gradually introduced to the child beginning at the age of 18 months. First, the child is provided with a potty chair; the child sits on the chair, fully clothed, for a few minutes each day. Next, the child sits on the potty chair without diapers. As the child becomes more interested in and comfortable with the potty chair, the child may be taken to the potty chair when his/her diaper is soiled. The diaper is then dropped into the potty chair to help the child learn the purpose of the chair. Next, the chair is placed in the child's play area, and he/she is told to use the potty, if need be. Once the child begins to use the potty chair, he/she is "graduated" to training pants; potty chair use is continued and encouraged. If the child does not make progress with the training, Brazelton recommends that training be stopped and resumed at a later time. Children are who are ready for toilet training will progress faster and be easier to train than those who are not yet ready.

Parents who desire a quicker method of toilet training may want to try Azrin and Foxx's *Toilet Training in Less Than a Day* program. As the title of the program suggests, this training method is designed to be implemented over the course of one day. The training is intense and involves providing the child with numerous opportunities to experience successful toileting. A toy doll that wets is used to model to the child the process of drinking and then urinating in the toilet. The child is encouraged to drink a large amount of liquids so that he/she will have repeated opportunities to practice using the toilet. If the child does wet his/her clothes during the training day, a mildly aversive consequence for wetting (helping clean up) is provided. Because of the potential for problems and side effects such as temper tantrums using the program, it is recommended that this program be applied only in consultation with a professional (Howe & Walker, 1992; Schroeder & Gordan, 2002).

Schroeder and Gordan (2002) outlined a somewhat modified approach to the child-oriented method. After determining that the child is ready for toilet training, parents begin tracking their child's toileting habits by checking his/her diaper on a regular basis. This helps parents know when the child is most likely to need to use the toilet. The child is then placed on the toilet at times when he/she is most likely to urinate or have a bowel movement. (See the later section on treatment of encopresis for more detailed information on "toilet sits.") If the child does urinate or defecate in the toilet, he/she is given a reinforcer. During this training time diapers are not used and accidents are handled in a matter-of-fact manner. Schroeder and Gordan indicate that when such a program is used, most children are successfully toilet trained within 2 to 4 weeks.

Most parents make it through the toilet-training phase without assistance from a medical or mental health professional. Typically it is only when a child continues to wet or have soiling accidents into the later preschool years, or when a child who was toilet trained resumes wetting or soiling, that a parent seeks professional help. Often parents will first seek assistance from their pediatrician (rather than a psychologist or other mental health professional). If a parent does first seek help from a mental health professional and has not consulted with his/her pediatrician, the mental health professional should refer the parent to a physician prior to implementing a behavioral treatment. Although enuresis and encopresis are rarely due to physical problems, such problems must be ruled out prior to the implementation of any psychosocial treatment.

Enuresis

As noted in Chapter 1, enuresis involves the voiding of urine in one's clothes during the daytime (diurnal enuresis) and/or while sleeping (nocturnal enuresis). To be diagnosed with enuresis, a child must be "having accidents" at least twice a week for at least 3 months (or there must be signs of significant distress or impairment in functioning; American Psychiatric Association, 1994). According to diagnostic guidelines in the DSM-IV, children must be at least 5 years of age to be diagnosed with enuresis. However, there is disagreement among clinicians regarding the appropriate cutoff age for diagnosis; some recommend a younger age and some, an older age. In addition, different cutoff ages may be appropriate for the different types of enuresis (diurnal vs. nocturnal). A younger age (3 or 4) may be a more appropriate cutoff for diurnal enuresis, while an older cutoff (6 or 7) may be more appropriate for nocturnal enuresis (Howe & Walker, 1992). Enuresis is also categorized as either primary or secondary. Children with primary enuresis have never achieved continuous bladder control, whereas children with secondary enuresis have been dry for some period of time (generally 6 months to 1 year) but then cease exhibiting bladder control (Howe & Walker, 1992).

Prevalence estimates for enuresis vary, with all estimates indicating a decline in prevalence as children age. It is estimated that approximately 15–20% of 5-year-olds wet the bed on a regular basis. This rate decreases to 5% of 10-year-olds and 2% of 12- to 14-year-olds (Howe & Walker, 1992). This decline with age is due, at least in part, to the fact that each year approximately 15% of children who wet the bed will cease to do so, even with no treatment (Forsythe & Redmond, 1974). Nocturnal enuresis is more common in boys than girls by about a 3:2 ratio (Mark & Frank, 1995). Diurnal enuresis is less common than nocturnal enuresis, with less than 3% of 6-year-olds meeting diagnostic criteria (Howe & Walker, 1992).

Before treatment for either diurnal or nocturnal enuresis is initiated, it is important to obtain a thorough understanding of the problem. Following a medical evaluation to rule out an organic cause, mental health professionals should obtain a full history of the child's wetting problems and any related toileting issues. In addition, the child's developmental history should be obtained. Parents also should be encouraged to track the child's wetting both initially, as part of the assessment process, as well as during treatment. (See Figures 5.1, 5.2, 5.3, and 5.4 for sample tracking sheets.)

Treatment of Diurnal Enuresis

Although there has been much research on nocturnal enuresis (bed-wetting), there is almost no research on the treatment of diurnal enuresis. If the child has never been dry during the day, it is likely that the child was never fully toilet trained. In this case, parents should consider reinstituting toilet-training procedures. If the child has been dry for some time but has begun to wet again, a modified version of Schroeder and Gordan's (2002) toilet-training approach is recommended. In addition to the toilet sits, parents should institute "dry-pant checks," in which they check the child's pants at certain times throughout the day and provide the child with a reinforcer if he/she is dry. When the child does wet, he/she should be required to assist with the cleanup, as appropriate for his/her age. Likely this will involve changing clothes and putting the wet clothes in a laundry hamper or other appropriate place. Schroeder and Gordan also suggest that children engage in "positive practice" activities, in which they practice walking to the bathroom and using the toilet from different locations (e.g., yard, different rooms in the house).

Treatment of Nocturnal Enuresis

Most parents will not implement treatment for nocturnal enuresis until early elementary school, so the discussion of this treatment applies more to kindergarten-age and older children. The standard psychosocial treatment for nocturnal enuresis is the "bell and pad" or "urine alarm" system. Medications such as imipramine or DDAVP may also be prescribed by the child's physician. Of these two medications, DDAVP is more effective and safer; thus its use is becoming more common and the use of imipramine is declining. Although DDAVP effectively alleviates nocturnal enuresis in many children, it is not a cure for it. Instead, children typically take DDAVP for a long period of time—likely they need to take it until the time they would naturally "outgrow" their bedwetting. The urine alarm has better long-term outcomes (Schulman, Colish, von Zuben, & Kodman-Jones, 2000) but is much more difficult for parents to use initially, and it can take several months for the child to become dry using this method.

Although the original urine alarm was, in fact, a bell and pad, today's alarms are more compact. The original alarm consisted of a pad that was connected to an alarm covering the bed; when the child began to wet, the moisture would set off sensors in the pad that caused the alarm to sound. The alarms in use today typically consist of snaps that are attached to the child's underwear. These are then connected to a small alarm box that can be worn on the child's wrist or shoulder. When the child wets, a connection is made between the snaps and the alarm sounds. Although there are several theories regarding why the alarm works,

DAYTIME WETTING LOG

Date	Time of wetting accident	Situation (what was happening)	Parent response to wetting

FIGURE 5.1. Daytime wetting log. From Gretchen A. Gimpel and Melissa L. Holland (2003). Copyright by The Guilford Press. Permission to photocopy this figure is granted to purchasers of this book for personal use only (see copyright page for details).

DAYTIME WETTING TREATMENT LOG

	Pant checks			Wetting accidents		
	Times	Dry (yes or no)	Reward (yes or no)	Times	Situation	Response
Sunday						
Monday						
Tuesday						
Wednesday						
Thursday						
Friday						
Saturday						

FIGURE 5.2. Daytime wetting treatment log. From Gretchen A. Gimpel and Melissa L. Holland (2003). Copyright by The Guilford Press. Permission to photocopy this figure is granted to purchasers of this book for personal use only (see copyright page for details).

NIGHTTIME WETTING LOG

	Bedtime	Wet? (yes or no) Record time(s) if known	Size of wet area	Parent response to wetting	Time awake
Sunday					
Monday					
Tuesday					
Wednesday					
Thursday					
Friday					
Saturday					

FIGURE 5.3. Nighttime wetting log. From Gretchen A. Gimpel and Melissa L. Holland (2003). Copyright by The Guilford Press. Permission to photocopy this figure is granted to purchasers of this book for personal use only (see copyright page for details).

NIGHTTIME WETTING AND ALARM USE LOG

	Bedtime	Wet? (yes or no) Record time(s)	Size of wet area	Alarm procedures follwed?(yes or no)	Reward given for following procedures or staying dry? (yes or no)	Time awake
Sunday						
Monday						
Tuesday						
Wednesday						
Thursday						
Friday						
Saturday						

FIGURE 5.4. Nighttime wetting and alarm use log. From Gretchen A. Gimpel and Melissa L. Holland (2003). Copyright by The Guilford Press. Permission to photocopy this figure is granted to purchasers of this book for personal use only (see copyright page for details).

none fully explains its effects. One theory is that the noise of the alarm is aversive to the child, so the child learns to wake to the sensation of a full bladder rather than wetting the bed. However, it appears that when children stop wetting the bed, many of them sleep through the night instead of waking up in the middle of the night to use the bathroom (Bonde, Anderson, & Rosenkilde, 1994). A variation on this theory suggests that children perceive both the alarm and waking as aversive consequences and thus learn to not wet the bed to avoid them.

The alarm is typically never used in isolation. Other treatment components, such as reinforcement for following the alarm procedures and cleanliness training (having the child assist with changing sheets and clothing following a wetting incident), are commonly part of a complete intervention package. In addition, methods such as *retention-control training,* in which the child drinks a large quantity of fluid and attempts to avoid urination as long as possible, and *overlearning,* in which the child consumes fluids prior to bedtime, also have been studied as added components to the alarm procedures. Although these add-on components may increase the effectiveness of the program (results are somewhat inconsistent on this matter), the alarm is clearly the most important treatment component (Howe & Walker, 1992).

Moisture alarms can be purchased from a variety of different companies and are sold under brand names such as Nytone, Sleep Dry, and Dri-Sleeper. Alarms cost approximately $50 to $75. Although parents can use the alarm without professional assistance, it is helpful for parents to consult with a behavior specialist when first setting up an alarm-based program. Following an initial consultation, parents should check in with the professional on an as-needed basis.

The use of the alarm should be discussed with both the parent and child present, and handouts on the use of the alarm should be provided. (See Figure 5.5 for a parent handout describing the use of the alarm and Figure 5.6 for a child handout that can be given to older children to read themselves or be read aloud to younger children.) It is important that both are agreeable to the use of the alarm, because both child and parent need to be active in the treatment procedures. Both should be shown how to attach the alarm, but the child should be responsible for attaching the alarm every night before he/she goes to bed. (The parent may want to check to make sure the alarm is attached appropriately.) When the alarm sounds, the parent should immediately wake up and go to the child's room—so it is important that the parent be able to hear the alarm. Placing a baby monitor in the child's room and/or leaving the bedroom doors of both rooms open can accomplish this component. When the alarm is first used, children often do not awaken to its sound. They should be instructed to listen for the alarm and to awaken if they hear it—but this often does not happen—so it is extremely important that the parent wake the child if he/she has not awakened on his/her own. Once the child is fully awake, he/she should detach the alarm, get up, go to the bathroom, and attempt to urinate in the toilet. Even if the child insists he/she no longer needs to go, this step should still be included. Afterward, the child should assist with any necessary clean-up (e.g., changing pajamas, changing the sheets). If the wet spot on the sheets is small, it is not necessary to change them during the night; instead, a towel can be placed over the spot. If the wet area is large (which is typical, at first), then the sheets should be changed. When the bed has been remade, the child should reattach the

TREATMENT OF BEDWETTING—USE OF THE ENURESIS ALARM: INSTRUCTIONS FOR PARENTS

The enuresis/moisture alarm can be an effective treatment for children who wet the bed. Alarms are sold under a variety of brand names, including Sleep Dry, Dri-Sleep, and Nytone. Most alarms today are small and consist of a sensor, worn in the child's underwear, which is hooked to a small alarm unit worn on the child's shoulder or wrist. When the child begins to wet, the sensor detects the moisture and the alarm sounds. For the alarm method to be successful, parents need to take an active role in treatment. Below are important guidelines.

At Night/During the Night

1. Make sure your child appropriately attaches the alarm each night before he/she goes to bed.
2. When the alarm sounds, immediately go to your child's room. Often the child will not awaken to the alarm at first, and he/she will need to be woken up by you.
3. Once your child is fully awake, have him/her detach the alarm and walk to the bathroom to finish urinating in the toilet. Even if your child says he/she no longer needs to urinate, he/she must at least try.
4. If the wet spot on the bed is large, assist your child in changing the bedding. (If the spot is small, consider placing a towel over it until the morning.) Your child also should change his/her clothing and place the wet clothing in an appropriate place (e.g., laundry hamper).
5. Have your child reattach the alarm and return to bed.
6. Repeat above procedures, as needed, throughout the night.

In the Morning

1. If your child did not wet, praise him/her for having a dry night.
2. If your child did not wet or if your child wet but he/she followed the alarm procedures appropriately, provide him/her with a small reward. It is important that rewards are given not just for staying dry but also for following the alarm procedures.
3. Record data on the progress chart.

Things to Remember

1. It is very important to remain neutral when your child wets. Do not become angry with your child or punish him/her for having a wet night. This program will work, but it takes time and patience.
2. When you first begin using the alarm your child may not wake up when the alarm goes off. This is not unusual and should not be cause for concern. However, it is important that you wake your child if this occurs. Thus, you need to be in a location where you can hear the alarm or use baby monitors (or a similar system) to allow you to hear the alarm.
3. Eventually your child will start waking on his/her own to the alarm. You will also begin to notice that the amount of urine in the bed has decreased until eventually there is just enough to set the alarm off. Dry nights will then begin to appear more frequently.
4. Your child should continue to wear the alarm until he/she has had 14 dry nights in a row. Following this you may discontinue use of the alarm. However, if your child resumes wetting the bed, immediately reinstate the use of the alarm and, again, continue using it until your child has 14 dry nights in a row.

FIGURE 5.5. Treatment of bedwetting—use of the enuresis alarm: Instructions for parents. From Gretchen A. Gimpel and Melissa L. Holland (2003). Copyright by The Guilford Press. Permission to photocopy this figure is granted to purchasers of this book for personal use only (see copyright page for details).

TREATMENT OF BEDWETTING—USE OF THE ENURESIS ALARM: INSTRUCTIONS FOR CHILDREN

The moisture alarm can help you learn to stop wetting the bed. The alarm does not shock you or hurt you in any way but will make a loud noise when you begin to wet the bed. The alarm will help you wake up during the night and use the toilet. For the alarm to work, it is important that you listen for it and wake up immediately when it goes off. Following the instructions below will help make the alarm successful and help you stop wetting the bed.

1. Hook up the alarm yourself each night. (If it is difficult to hook up, ask your mother or father for help.)

2. When the alarm sounds, wake up and stop wetting. It is important to do this as soon as you hear the alarm.

3. After you wake up, disconnect the alarm.

4. Go to the bathroom and at least try to go in the toilet.

5. Put on clean underwear and pajamas, change your sheets (with your parents' help) and reconnect the alarm.

6. If the alarm goes off again during the night, repeat these same steps.

7. In the morning, mark on your chart whether you were wet or dry.

8. Use the alarm every night until you are dry for 14 nights in a row.

It may take a little while for you to stop wetting the bed completely. Don't become discouraged—just keep using the alarm!

FIGURE 5.6. Treatment of bedwetting—use of the enuresis alarm: instructions for children. From Gretchen A. Gimpel and Melissa L. Holland (2003). Copyright by The Guilford Press. Permission to photocopy this figure is granted to purchasers of this book for personal use only (see copyright page for details).

alarm and return to bed. If the alarm sounds again during the night, these same procedures should be repeated. During these nighttime proceedings it is essential that the parent not become angry with, or punish, the child. The parent should assist the child matter-of-factly with the alarm procedures.

In the morning, the child should receive a small reward if he/she stayed dry during the night or if he/she followed the alarm procedures correctly. Because it will take some time for the child to begin to have dry nights consistently, the child should be rewarded simply for following the procedures correctly. If these procedures are followed on a nightly basis, the child should become dry. The child also should track his/her wet and dry nights on a chart so that progress can be seen. If the child was dry during the night, the parent should praise the child for staying dry, but if the child was wet, the parent should not be discouraging or negative. Instead the parent should simply praise the child for following the alarm procedures (if the child did so) and perhaps make a matter-of-fact comment such as, "Even though you wet last night, you did a great job following the alarm procedures. Maybe you'll be dry tonight."

The alarm does not produce immediate effects; in fact, it is not unusual for it to take several months for the child to become consistently dry during the night. One of the first indicators of progress is that the wet spots in the bed become smaller. This decrease occurs because the child begins to awaken more quickly to the alarm and stops voiding until he/she gets to the bathroom. The alarm should be used until the child has 14 dry nights in a row. Following this accomplishment, the use of the alarm can be discontinued. However, if the child begins to wet again, use of the alarm should be reinstated immediately and should continue until the child again has 14 consecutive dry nights.

Encopresis

Encopresis involves soiling in inappropriate places, such as clothing, at least once a month for at least 3 months (American Psychiatric Association, 1994). Encopresis is typically due to severe constipation and is referred to as *retentive* encopresis. However, a small portion of children with encopresis (5–20%) exhibit nonretentive encopresis. This category includes children who were never fully toilet trained, those with some type of fear related to toileting, those who engage in manipulative soiling, and those with irritable bowel syndrome (Kuhn et al., 1999). To receive a diagnosis of encopresis, a child must be at least 4 years old. However, it is not uncommon for children under the age of 4 to exhibit problems such as refusing to use the toilet. Children who exhibit toileting refusal are at risk of developing encopresis due to constipation (Brooks et al., 2000).

When a child is encopretic a medical evaluation should be conducted to rule out the possibility of any organic etiology. Encopresis rarely has an organic etiology; about 95% of the cases of retentive encopresis and 99% of the cases of nonretentive encopresis do not have an organic etiology (Kuhn et al., 1999); however, it is important to confirm this absence before proceeding with a behavioral treatment.

In children with retentive encopresis, the encopresis is a result of extreme constipation. For variety of reasons, children may not have regular bowel movements. When a child does not have a bowel movement in response to the need to do so, the fecal material returns to the colon. This fecal material then becomes hardened, which makes it more difficult and painful for the child to pass. As the child becomes more and more constipated, fecal material becomes impacted in the colon. In addition, the muscles around the colon become stretched; as a result, the child is unable to feel the need to have a bowel movement and is unable to pass bowel movements effectively. Typically, fluid leaks out around the impaction, producing some soiling. Children with retentive encopresis often do not know when this leaking occurs and therefore are not aware of the soiling. In addition to this leakage, occasionally large fecal masses are expelled (Schroeder & Gordan, 2002; Walker, 1995).

Children with nonretentive encopresis are not constipated, so impaction of feces is not a problem for them. They typically have consistent bowel movements and stools that are normal in size. In addition, whereas children with retentive encopresis may complain of abdominal pain, such complaints are not typical in children with nonretentive encopresis (Kuhn et al., 1999).

Treatment of Retentive Encopresis

The typical treatment program for retentive encopresis, which has been demonstrated to be effective (Brooks et al., 2000), involves a combination of medical procedures and behavioral interventions. As mentioned above, it is important that children with encopresis receive a medical evaluation prior to treatment. In addition to ruling out an organic etiology, the physician can discuss any medical interventions that should occur with the parents. Often, because the child's colon is very impacted with fecal material, it is necessary to administer a series of enemas to clear out this material. Enemas should be administered under the direction of a physician and prior to the implementation of behavioral interventions, as these will likely be less successful if the child is still severely impacted. The physician may also recommend stool softeners or laxatives to help ensure regular bowel movements.

Parents also should receive instruction regarding appropriate dietary modifications; children with encopresis need to consume an appropriate amount of fiber. The consumption of fruits and vegetables should be encouraged. In addition, wheat germ or bran may be sprinkled on food as a supplement. Parents also should be encouraged to increase their child's fluid intake and to cut down the child's consumption of dairy products, if it is high. It may be beneficial for the family to consult with a nutritionist who can assist parents in making appropriate dietary modifications.

The behavioral component of an encopresis treatment programs involves the implementation of regular "toilet sits" as well as rewards for producing a bowel movement in the toilet. Toilet sits encourage the child to use the toilet and also help the child establish a routine of using the toilet when he/she is most likely to have a bowel movement. Toilet sits are a key component to treatment programs; children who do not engage in the prescribed toilet sits are more likely to show little or no improvement (Brooks et al., 2000). Children should engage in two to four toilet sits per day, at times when they are most likely to have a bowel movement (e.g., soon after waking up in the morning; after mealtimes). During a toilet sit, the child remains on the toilet for 5–10 minutes. Toilet sits should be fun and enjoyable; the child should be given a book or toy with which to play or be allowed to listen to music while in the bathroom. Obviously, the toilet needs to be comfortable for the child, and his/her feet should reach the floor (parents can use either a potty chair or provide a stool on which the child can rest his/her feet). If the child is successful at having a bowel movement (i.e., the child has a bowel movement consisting of approximately a quarter to a half a cup of fecal material), he/she receives a reward. In addition, parents should also institute "clean pants checks" several times a day and give a reward to the child if he/she has not had a soiling accident. Soiled pants should be treated matter-of-factly; the child (with assistance from a parent as needed) should be required to wash his/her underwear in the sink or bathtub, then clean him/herself and get redressed. Parents should make sure not to nag or punish their child for soiling—a matter-of-fact tone is far more effective (Howe & Walker, 1992; Schroeder & Gordan, 2002). (See Figure 5.7 for a parent handout detailing the treatment of encopresis, and Figure 5.8 for a treatment log for parents to use in tracking treatment progress.)

Treatment of Toileting Refusal/Nonretentive Encopresis

As noted above, retentive encopresis is the more common type of encopresis. However, children may also be encopretic for reasons other than constipation. In young children, particularly, refusing to use the toilet may become a problem. Children who exhibit toileting refusal simply refuse to sit on the toilet. This refusal may be due to the child's negative associations with the bathroom and the toilet due to past painful bowel movements, or other negative toileting experiences.

If the child exhibits fear in relation to the bathroom or toileting, more positive stimuli need to be associated with toileting procedures. One way to help the child learn to associate the bathroom and the toilet with positive stimuli is through the use of planned, positive toilet sits (Kuhn et al., 1999). These sits are similar to those described above; however, the initial purpose of these sits is not to encourage the child to have a bowel movement in the toilet but to simply help reduce the child's anxiety about the toilet. Thus, during these initial sits, the child can wear a diaper or other clothing. Initially these sits should be fairly brief in time (perhaps less than 1 minute), but the time should be increased as the child becomes more comfortable. As with the toilet sits described above, the child should be comfortable on the toilet, and the setting and atmosphere should be fun; the child should be encouraged to listen to music, bring books into the bathroom, etc. In addition, these sits should be associated with positive parent–child interactions. Parents should make sure not to nag or scold their child during this time but instead should interact with him/her in a positive, child-directed manner.

In some instances, the child may be so resistant to scheduled toilet sits that these will have to be shaped more gradually. In this situation Kuhn et al. (1999) recommend that parents begin by modeling appropriate toileting behavior. After this step, parents should engage their child in fun activities in the bathroom (or close to the bathroom). For example,

TREATMENT GUIDELINES FOR CHILDREN WITH ENCOPRESIS

Encopresis (fecal soiling) is defined as a child over the age of 4 having a bowel movement in inappropriate places (e.g., clothing). Approximately 1–2% of children have this problem, and it is more common in boys than girls. Encopresis is most often the result of chronic constipation. Children who become severely constipated will have leakage of fecal material but be unaware of it. It is important to remember that, in most cases, the child is not soiling intentionally and cannot control the soiling response. By following the guidelines below, you should see results within a month or 2.

1. Prior to implementing other treatment procedures, take your child to his/her physician for an examination. The following steps will not be successful if the child is still severely constipated and has impacted fecal material. Your child's physician may suggest administering an enema to "clean out" your child's bowels. The physician also may instruct you to give your child mineral oil and/or laxatives to keep material moving through the intestinal system. It is important to follow your physician's recommendations carefully.

2. Have your child engage in regular toilet sits. Approximately 2–4 times a day, schedule 5–10-minute toilet sits at times when your child is most likely to have a bowel movement (e.g., soon after waking in the morning, 15–20 minutes after meals). Make sure that the bathroom and the toilet are comfortable for the child. Your child's feet should be able to rest flatly on the floor or a stool, and the toilet seat should be sized appropriately. Allow your child to bring a favorite toy or book into the bathroom so that he/she can engage in a pleasant activity while sitting on the toilet.

3. Reward your child for appropriate bowel movements. If your child has a bowel movement (approximately one-quarter to one-half cup in size) in the toilet, provide a small reward to him/her. It is a good idea to have different rewards available, so that your child does not tire of the same reward. Allowing your child to draw a reward coupon out of a bag or spin a game-wheel to determine what reward he/she gets can be fun for the child. Rewards do not have to be large and can include extra time with a parent, a special dessert, being allowed to watch extra TV, etc. Rewards should be given to the child as immediately as possible (and at least within the same day).

4. Conduct pants checks. Several times throughout the day, check your child's pants. If he/she has soiled, he/she should be responsible for cleanup. Your child should rinse and wash out his/her underwear and pants, bathe quickly, and put on clean clothes. (You may assist with these steps if your child is not able to complete the cleanup process on his/her own.) If your child has not soiled when these pant checks are conducted, give him/her a small reward.

5. Ensure that your child is getting adequate nutrition. For regular bowel movements to occur, it is important that your child's diet include adequate amounts of fiber. Make sure your child eats plenty of fruits and vegetables, and consider sprinkling bran or wheat germ on foods. In addition, dairy products should be limited (although not cut out completely). The combination of fiber, water, and regular exercise will promote regular bowel movements. You may find it helpful to consult with a nutritionist who can help you modify your child's diet.

6. Record your child's progress. You and your child should keep a chart of your child's bowel movements, toilet sits, and pant checks. Keeping a chart will help you both see progress as well as stick to the treatment plan.

FIGURE 5.7. Treatment guidelines for children with encopresis. From Gretchen A. Gimpel and Melissa L. Holland (2003). Copyright by The Guilford Press. Permission to photocopy this figure is granted to purchasers of this book for personal use only (see copyright page for details).

ENCOPRESIS TREATMENT LOG

	Toilet sits			Pant checks	
	Times	Bowel movement (yes or no)	Reward (yes or no)	Times	Clean (yes or no)	Reward (yes or no)
Sunday						
Monday						
Tuesday						
Wednesday						
Thursday						
Friday						
Saturday						

FIGURE 5.8. Encopresis treatment log. From Gretchen A. Gimpel and Melissa L. Holland (2003). Copyright by The Guilford Press. Permission to photocopy this figure is granted to purchasers of this book for personal use only (see copyright page for details).

parents may play the child's favorite game with him/her in the doorway to the bathroom. These fun activities are then gradually moved closer to the toilet, and eventually the parent has the child engage in these activities while sitting on the toilet.

Once the child has overcome his/her toileting "fear" and is having regular and normal bowel movements, parents can shift to working on training the child to have bowel movements in the toilet. Parents should instigate regular toilet sits (in which the child is no longer wearing a diaper) two to four times a day, as described above. It is important that the positive activities initiated during the toilet sits be continued and that the child be provided with incentives for having a bowel movement in the toilet (Kuhn et al., 1999).

FEEDING/EATING PROBLEMS AND INTERVENTIONS

Feeding disorders include an array of behaviors that involve the refusal to eat certain foods or the actual inability to eat certain foods. These problems may be due to organic causes, such as metabolic or neuromuscular problems, or behavioral/psychosocial issues (Babbitt et al., 1994). Feeding disorders are seen in both typically developing young children as well as children with developmental disabilities and medical conditions. Although feeding problems are considered to be common in typically developing children, with estimates ranging widely from 2–45% (Kedesdy & Budd, 1998), they are thought to be even more common in children with developmental delays (Kerwin, 1999). Most feeding problems are not long-lasting, and parents may never seek treatment. In a smaller subset of children, feeding problems may be persistent and require more focused interventions.

Although there are a variety of feeding disorders children may exhibit (some of which are due to complex medical complications) this chapter focuses on the more common, everyday variety that parents may encounter with their preschool- and kindergarten-age children: "picky" eaters who eat only a limited number of food items as well as those who refuse to eat. Brief discussions of pica (in which children consume nonfood objects) and rumination (in which children repeatedly regurgitate and rechew their food) also are included. In addition to these difficulties, many feeding problems involve children who display inappropriate behavior at mealtimes (e.g., throwing temper tantrums). For children with this type of problem, the guidelines outlined in Chapter 3 (for the treatment of externalizing problems) should be followed.

Treatment of Typical Feeding Problems

The primary interventions for feeding disorders involve behavioral methods. No matter what the initial cause of the problem, children with feeding problems often are reinforced for their inappropriate feeding behaviors. For example, parents may comment on or attempt to correct their child's spitting out of food (although this attention is typically negative, it is often reinforcing to the child); parents may give their child the foods he/she prefers if the child becomes upset when given other foods; or parents may allow their child to leave the feeding situation when he/she misbehaves (Babbitt et al., 1994). Given that it is often the reinforcement of inappropriate eating behaviors that either causes or exacerbates feeding problems, it is logical that behavioral interventions are the most common and effective interventions for these difficulties. The behavioral principles used (and supported by research) are fairly straightforward: positive reinforcement for appropriate feeding behaviors, and the removal of positives or the application of mildly aversive consequences for inappropriate behaviors.

Because feeding disorders can have an organic component, a child with an ongoing feeding problem should first receive a medical evaluation. Behavioral interventions may still be part of the treatment package, but other interventions also may be appropriate. For the typically developing child, feeding problems have more of an environmental component, and assessment of the feeding problems should focus on determining the antecedents and consequences for both appropriate and inappropriate feeding behaviors (assuming that the child has received a medical evaluation and has been found to have no medical problems). Specific behaviors that the child engages in should be identified and operationally defined, and the settings surrounding these behaviors should be clear. In addition, the clinician should inquire about parental responses to the child's behaviors, foods the child likes/does not like, etc. (see Table 5.1 for interview/guidelines; Babbitt et al., 1994; Kedesdy & Budd, 1998). This assessment information helps the clinician develop an intervention program that targets the contingencies that are maintaining the feeding difficulties.

Environmental changes regarding mealtime may be necessary to improve the child's eating patterns. Parents should make sure they provide portions that are appropriately sized to the child's developmental level and weight. In addition, the child should be com-

---

TABLE 5.1. Interview Questions for Parents Regarding Their Child's Eating Problems

Describe the specific problem behaviors your child exhibits in relation to eating.

How long have these problems been going on?

What have you tried previously to decrease these problem behaviors? What has been the most successful? What has not worked?

How long does your child engage in eating (e.g., how long does your child stay at the dinner table)? What portion of a meal does your child generally eat?

Does your child feed him/herself? If not, who does? If so, any problems with this?

What times of day does your child eat? (Include all instances of eating—snacks and meals.)

What does your child typically eat in these instances? Where does the eating occur?

What foods does your child like/dislike? Are there certain textures, types of foods, etc., for which your child has a preference? What foods are routinely not eaten, spit out, etc.?

Are there certain settings, foods, etc., that are likely to prompt your child's feeding problems? Please describe these.

When your child engages in problem eating behaviors, what do you do?

Give an example of a recent interaction you had with your child related to feeding. Describe the setting, your child's behaviors, and your actions.

Describe a typical mealtime in your house.

Do you have any other behavioral concerns about your child?

Source. Babbitt et al. (1994) and Kedesday and Budd (1998).

fortably seated at mealtimes, and distractions (such as TV) should be reduced or eliminated (Kedesdy & Budd, 1998).

Giving positive attention for appropriate feeding behaviors is one of the most common interventions recommended for feeding problems. When the child is eating appropriately, the parent praises him/her. When the child is not eating appropriately, the parent is instructed to ignore him/her for a brief period of time, attending to the child again only when he/she resumes appropriate eating behaviors. (If the child's inappropriate behaviors are particularly severe or lengthy, this method will need to be combined with other methods.) At the initial stages of the intervention, positive reinforcement may be provided for each instance of appropriate eating behavior. As the child begins to engage in more and more appropriate eating behaviors, the reinforcement provided should gradually be decreased (Babbitt et al., 1994; Kerwin, 1999; Linscheid, Budd, & Rasnake, 1995).

In addition to using social attention to encourage eating, preferred foods may be used as rewards. This intervention, based on the Premack principle (using a high probability behavior to reinforce a low probability behavior), is commonly recommended along with social attention. In such an intervention, the child would be allowed to have several bites of pizza (a highly preferred food) after eating several bites of carrots (a nonpreferred food). Tangible reinforcers also can be used to help shape appropriate eating behaviors. Children may earn special privileges (e.g., inviting a friend over, staying up later) for engaging in appropriate eating behavior.

In addition to providing positive reinforcers to the child for appropriate eating behaviors, consequences may be implemented for inappropriate eating behaviors (e.g., spitting out food, refusing food, throwing a tantrum). Time-out is one negative consequence that may be used. However, for children who find eating to be aversive, time-out may simply be seen as a method of escaping something they do not want to do in the first place (i.e., eat). If time-out is used it is important to include a strong positive reinforcer for eating, per se, and for appropriate eating behavior (Babbitt et al., 1994; O'Brien, Repp, Willliams, & Christophersen, 1991). Other common negative consequences for inappropriate eating behavior include the removal of preferred food items or the loss of desired privileges (Kedesdy & Budd, 1998; Linscheid et al., 1995). (See Figure 5.9 for a parent handout that summarizes these treatment options.)

In typically developing children, providing positive reinforcement for appropriate eating behaviors and negative consequences for inappropriate eating behaviors likely will be sufficient to overcome any problems in this area. However, in developmentally delayed children and some children with more severe feeding problems, additional methods may be necessary. These include methods of physical guidance, such as jaw prompting, in which the clinician or parent puts food in the child's mouth while holding the chin with his/her thumb and index finger. After the child chews and swallows the food, the child's jaw is released (O'Brien et al., 1991). Punishment techniques include spraying lemon juice into a child's mouth following inappropriate eating behaviors, and overcorrection (e.g., having a child repeatedly cleanup after spitting out food). These more aversive techniques are not recommended, unless the positive reinforcement and milder versions of punishment (e.g., time-out) are not successful (Kedesdy & Budd, 1998). With the vast majority of normally developing children, these aversive techniques will not be needed.

SOLUTIONS TO MEALTIME PROBLEMS: GUIDELINES FOR PARENTS

Difficult behaviors at mealtimes are common in young children. Typically these problems are not long-lasting and are not an indicator of more serious problems. However, before implementing any of the techniques outlined below, you should have your child evaluated by a physician to rule out any possible medical cause of your child's eating difficulties.

"Picky" eating is the most common eating problem exhibited by young children. Picky eaters include children who eat only a limited number of foods and/or very small portions of foods. The picky eater may have his/her favorite foods (e.g., grapes and bananas) and refuse to eat other foods, and/or the picky eater may eat unusually small portions of food. These children also frequently exhibit problem behaviors at mealtimes. They may whine about the food presented to them, spit out food, or engage in tantrum throwing or other inappropriate behaviors.

Below are guidelines to help you increase your child's appropriate eating behaviors.

1. **Create a pleasant mealtime environment.** It is important that the environment surrounding eating be pleasant for the child and focused on eating and positive family interactions. Your child should be seated comfortably at mealtimes, and distractions should be reduced (e.g., turn off the TV). In addition, make sure the foods and portions you are giving to your child are appropriate for his/her age, size, and developmental level. If you are unsure about appropriate portion size, consult with a pediatrician or a dietician.
2. **Provide positive verbal attention for appropriate eating behaviors.** When your child engages in appropriate eating behaviors (e.g., eating politely, not whining), praise for these behaviors (e.g., "I really like how you're eating the food on your plate and talking nicely to us.").
3. **Use preferred foods as reinforcers.** Although it is not important that your child eat a wide variety of foods, you will likely want your child to accept and eat the foods your typically have for dinner. To increase the number of foods your child eats, try pairing a food your child finds very desirable with a food your child is less sure about. For example, if your child really likes grapes (not a typical dinner item at your household) but does not like peas (a typical dinner item), let him/her know that he/she can have some grapes after he/she eats some peas; the grapes reinforce the child's willingness to eat the peas.
4. **Set up a reward program.** Set up rules for mealtimes and give your child a reward if he/she follows these rules. Rules might include: "No whining about the food, eat at least half of what is on your plate [assuming portion size is correct], and no spitting out food." If your child follows these rules during the meal, he/she is allowed to choose from a special "treat jar" that contains a number of items that he/she finds reinforcing (e.g., small toys, stickers, passes for special time with Mom or Dad). As with any reward program, it is important that you keep the expectations reasonable (e.g., do not expect a child who is eating one-eighth of the meal to start eating all of the meal) and that the rewards be items your child truly enjoys. It is a good idea to put in new rewards on a regular basis so that your child does not become bored with the available rewards.
5. **Provide consequences for inappropriate eating behaviors.** If the positive approach alone does not work, or if your child is engaging in several acting-out behaviors (and is not just refusing to eat), consider implementing consequences for these inappropriate behaviors. Consequences may include a loss of a certain privilege for the rest of the day (e.g., no watching TV), not receiving preferred food items, or time-out. However, be careful about the use of time-out for a child who is refusing to eat. This child may find eating aversive and may engage in behaviors to "escape" the eating situation. Thus, for this child, time-out can actually reinforce the problem behaviors.

FIGURE 5.9. Solutions to mealtime problems: guidelines for parents. From Gretchen A. Gimpel and Melissa L. Holland (2003). Copyright by The Guilford Press. Permission to photocopy this figure is granted to purchasers of this book for personal use only (see copyright page for details).

Pica

Pica refers to the eating of non-nutritive substances, including paint, cloth, sand, etc. It is relatively common for infants toddlers to eat non-food substances occasionally. This behavior does not necessarily imply the presence of pica, which should not be diagnosed unless the behavior is inappropriate for the child's developmental level and persists for at least 1 month (American Psychiatric Association, 1994). Because pica can be dangerous to the child (e.g., ingestion of lead paint), it should be treated. As with other feeding problems, behavioral interventions are the most recommended form of treatment. Discrimination training may be needed (i.e., teaching the child to be able to identify food and nonfood items), especially for children with developmental delays. In a treatment program for pica, children should earn reinforcers for eating appropriate food substances and receive a mild punishment for eating nonfood substances. Time-out can be an effective punishment. In addition, the application of water mist or lemon juice has been found effective (Kedesdy & Budd, 1998; Motta & Basile, 1998). Overcorrection (as discussed in the previous section) also has been used, with success, in several treatment programs; consequences used following pica behaviors have included a period of tooth brushing or face washing as well as cleaning/tidying of the room (Bell & Stein, 1992).

Rumination

Rumination involves repeatedly regurgitating and rechewing food. This behavior typically emerges after a period of normal functioning; it must occur for at least 1 month for the child to receive a diagnosis. Children with rumination disorder regurgitate partially digested food into their mouths (with no associated nausea, etc.) and then spit out or rechew the food. The disorder is most common in infants but is also diagnosed in older children, particularly those with mental retardation (American Psychiatric Association, 1994). Rumination is voluntary and actually appears to be pleasurable to the child engaging in the behavior. Children with rumination are at-risk for a number of problems, including social difficulties as well as health problems (e.g., malnutrition, dehydration, dental problems); thus treatment is typically recommended (Kedesdy & Budd, 1998). As with the other feeding disorders, behavioral interventions are commonly applied. These include reinforcement for nonruminating eating behavior or reinforcement of a response that does not allow the child to engage in the ruminating behavior. For example, if a child uses his/her finger to induce rumination, reinforce the child for another activity that requires his/her hands (e.g., drawing, building with blocks, holding a utensil correctly).

Punishment also has been incorporated into these behavioral treatment programs. Techniques used have included mild punishments, such as time-out or the application of lemon juice, as well as more severe punishments (e.g., electric shock), which should not be administered on an outpatient basis (or at all, many would argue). In addition to the standard behavior interventions, "therapeutic nurturing" has been a recommended (although not well-studied) procedure; it involves the child receiving extensive noncontingent social attention from caregivers (i.e., providing attention that is not preceded by the performance of a specified behavior). Altering the feeding rate by giving repeated smaller portions of food, rather than one larger portion all at once, as well as satiation (allowing the child to eat unlimited amounts of food during mealtimes) also have been used to treat rumination (Kedesdy & Budd, 1998). Although all of these techniques have received some empirical support, the research on these techniques (particularly with young, non-delayed children) is still quite limited.

SLEEP PROBLEMS

Preschool-age children may exhibit a variety of difficulties related to sleep. The most common problems include resistance to going to bed and frequent waking during the night. Other common problems include nightmares, night terrors, and sleep talking and sleep walking. About 25% of 5-year-old children have some type of sleep disturbance (Mindell, 1993). These problems will be temporary for some children but will persist over time for others. Persistence of sleep problems is particularly likely to occur when children begin exhibiting sleep problems at an early age (Mindell, 1993).

Sleep problems obviously may be cause for concern for parents who themselves are losing sleep because of their child's difficulties. Sleep problems also may have more detrimental consequences. Although there is little research on the effects of sleep loss in children (particularly young children), studies have demonstrated that sleep loss can result in cognitive impairments (e.g., impaired school performance, impaired creativity and abstract reasoning) as well as increased behavior problems such as irritability and overactivity (Stores, 2001). Thus treating sleep problems may have the added benefit of reducing other behavior problems and improving school performance. In addition, child sleep problems may cause problems for parents that lead to marital difficulties, and may be a risk factor for abuse (Kerr & Jowett, 1994). Because sleep problems can have an impact on other problems commonly seen in preschool age-children (e.g., general externalizing problems), clinicians should routinely ask about sleep-related issues in any initial interview with the parents of a referred child.

Prior to developing an intervention for a child's sleep problems, it is important to conduct a thorough assessment of the sleep-related problems. An interview with the child's parents (see Table 5.2) as well as logs of the child's sleep problems (see Figures 5.10 and 5.11) are important to obtain. Information on the child's bedtime routine and the parents' response to the child if he/she awakens during the night is particularly salient. Often parents unwittingly reinforce their child's sleep problems by immediately responding when the child awakens during the night. Thus the child learns (and comes to expect) that when he/she cries, his/her parents will respond. Most young children do not sleep continuously through the night but awaken several times. If parents immediately respond when the child awakens and stay with the child until he/she falls back asleep, the child never learns to self-soothe and instead becomes dependent on his/her parents to return to sleep. For most children who exhibit sleep problems involving nighttime waking, it is not a problem of staying asleep but a problem of initiating sleep (France, Henderson, & Hudson, 1996).

TABLE 5.2. Interview Questions for Parents Regarding Their Child's Sleep Behaviors

Describe your child's current sleep pattern and sleep difficulties (e.g., what occurs and when).

How long have these difficulties been present?

Did anything (e.g., birth of a sibling, starting daycare, marital arguments) precipitate these problems?

Is there anything that makes your child's sleep problems better or worse?

What do you do in response to your child's wakings/difficulties falling asleep?

Describe your typical bedtime routine with your child, including who puts child to bed, when, where (e.g., child's room, parents' room), how long you stay with your child, etc.

What happens before beginning the bedtime routine?

When does your child wake up in the morning? Does your child wake up on his/her own? If not, who awakens your child and how?

Does your child awaken during the night? If so, describe what happens (how often child awakens, what you do, etc.).

Does your child have nightmares, engage in sleepwalking, wet the bed, or have any other sleep-related problems? If so, describe.

Source. Stores (2001).

Problems Initiating Sleep

Difficulty initiating sleep, although generally not considered diagnosable, can cause problems for parents and has been the focus of much of the literature on sleep problems in children. Typically children with this problem refuse to go to bed or engage in lengthy stalling behaviors. In addition, if the child awakens during the night, he/she often has difficulty getting back to sleep. Although night wakings generally decrease from the infant/toddler years to the preschool years, they still cause difficulties for a number of preschool-age children, with prevalence estimates ranging from 5–30% (Mindell, 1993, 1996; Stores, 2001). Treatment for problems initiating sleep focus on behavioral interventions such as establishing bedtime routines, extinction, and night wakings. These procedures, which are described below, all have some empirical support (Mindell, 1993, 1999). A parent handout summarizing these interventions is included in Figure 5.12.

Developing Bedtime Routines

Developing bedtime routines can be effective in reducing problematic sleep-related behaviors. When first developing a routine, parents are instructed to move the child's bedtime gradually to the time when the child naturally becomes sleepy. In addition, parents are instructed to put in place a series of relaxing activities that are engaged in prior to this bedtime. These activities may include taking a bath, reading a story, or listening to soft music (Kuhn & Weidinger, 2000; Mindell, 1999). This bedtime routine, as well as the child's bedroom/sleeping environment, should help set the stage for sleep to occur, and the routine should assist the child in associating his/her bed with nonstimulating, restful behaviors (Stores, 2001). Parents should ensure that the child's sleep environment is conducive to sleep. The bedroom should be quiet and the temperature adequately controlled (not too hot or too cold). In addition, the child's bed should be comfortable and age-

SLEEP CHART

	Wake-up time	Nap time(s)	Time begin bedtime routine	Time in bed	Time asleep	Times wakes up during night
Sunday						
Monday						
Tuesday						
Wednesday						
Thursday						
Friday						
Saturday						

FIGURE 5.10. Sleep chart. From Gretchen A. Gimpel and Melissa L. Holland (2003). Copyright by The Guilford Press. Permission to photocopy this figure is granted to purchasers of this book for personal use only (see copyright page for details).

NIGHTTIME WAKINGS CHART

Day	Time awake	Your response	Time back to sleep
Example:			
Sunday	11 P.M.	Rocked, gave drink	11:30 P.M.
Sunday	2 A.M.	Ignored	2:15 A.M.
Sunday	4 A.M.	Got in bed with	4:20 A.M.

FIGURE 5.11. Nighttime wakings chart. From Gretchen A. Gimpel and Melissa L. Holland (2003). Copyright by The Guilford Press. Permission to photocopy this figure is granted to purchasers of this book for personal use only (see copyright page for details).

138

SOLUTIONS TO SLEEP PROBLEMS

If your child seems to be resistant to going to bed (he/she cries, whines, asks for one more drink, etc.), or if your child frequently awakens during the night and cries until you comfort him/her, there are several treatment options that can reduce these problems. Prior to implementing any of these programs, make sure that your child has an appropriate bedtime routine. This routine should involve activities that are relaxing (e.g., reading a book) and set the stage for sleep. You should work to establish a standard bedtime for your child and begin the routine 15–30 minutes prior to that bedtime.

Complete Ignoring

1. Put your child to bed following his/her bedtime routine.
2. When you child cries after being put to bed and during the night, do not respond.

Gradual Ignoring

1. Put your child to bed following his/her bedtime routine.
2. If your child cries after being put to bed or during the night, immediately check on him/her.
3. Initially spend slightly less time than you had been previously spending with your child when he/she awoke during the night. (For example, if you had been spending an average of 30 minutes with your child, reduce that to 25 minutes.)
4. Once the preset attending time is up, leave the child and do not return. (If the child falls back to sleep and again awakens, repeat the procedure.)
5. Over time, reduce the amount of time you spend with your child during these attending periods.

Brief Checks

1. Put your child to bed following his/her bedtime routine.
2. If your child cries after being put to bed or awakens during the night crying, briefly check on your child every 5–10 minutes until he/she stops crying.
3. During these checks, do not give extended attention to your child. Simply give your child a pat on the back or head, retuck the child's blankets, or say "good-night." Once this is done, leave the room.
4. Over time, as your child begins to sleep longer, increase the time between checks.

Gradual Withdrawal of Parent

Prior to beginning this program, put a bed for yourself in your child's room.

1. Put your child to bed following his/her bedtime routine.
2. If your child cries, lie down on your bed and pretend to be asleep.
3. While you are pretending to be asleep, ignore the child's crying.
4. Once your child has fallen asleep, leave the room.
5. If your child cries during the night, return to the child's room and your bed there. Pretend to be asleep and ignore the child's crying. Again, leave when the child falls back to sleep.
6. After one week, return to sleeping in your own room and ignore your child's crying.

(continued)

FIGURE 5.12. Solutions to sleep problems. From Gretchen A. Gimpel and Melissa L. Holland (2003). Copyright by The Guilford Press. Permission to photocopy this figure is granted to purchasers of this book for personal use only (see copyright page for details).

Scheduled Wakings

1. Keep a chart noting when your child typically awakens during the night.
2. Put your child to bed following his/her bedtime routine.
3. Awaken your child 15–30 minutes before he/she typically awakens during the night.
4. After waking the child, interact with him/her as you would when he/she awoke on his/her own during the night.
5. Gradually lengthen the amount of time you wait before awakening your child.

Important Points to Keep in Mind

When you are using a method that includes ignoring your child, the child's behavior typically gets worse before it gets better. This is referred to as an "extinction burst." Your child is used to getting your attention and he/she will try harder (through longer, louder crying, etc.) when you first start ignoring the behavior. It is very important that you continue to ignore the child (as defined by the plan you are following). Attending to increases in crying will likely only make it more difficult to decrease this behavior.

When using a method that involves ignoring, initially you may see improvement but then a return to the crying. Do not be discouraged by this turn of events. Again, the child is used to getting your attention and is testing you to see what will happen. Continue to follow the program's stipulations for ignoring your child's problematic behaviors.

appropriate, and a night-light should be allowed, if desired by the child. Once the child is going to bed without significant problems, the bedtime and its associated routine can be gradually moved back to the time desired by the parents (Kuhn & Weidinger, 2000; Mindell, 1999).

Although it is important for the child to associate bed and bedtime with relaxing activities, clinicians should ensure that parents do not inadvertently establish routines that are nonconducive to the child settling him/herself. For example, parents should be discouraged from rocking their child to sleep, providing the child with a bottle until he/she falls asleep, etc. If such activities become routine, it may become difficult for the child to fall back to sleep without the assistance of these activities/objects. Reducing these parent-dependent cues at bedtime also can make it more likely that a child will fall back asleep on his/her own after waking during the night (Stores, 2001).

Extinction-Based Interventions

Extinction of the undesired response, through ignoring, is one of the most common recommendations made to parents of children with sleep problems. This technique, which involves having the parent ignore the child after putting him/her to bed, has been demonstrated to be effective in reducing sleep problems (Mindell, 1999). Extinction is based on the idea that the child exhibiting sleep problems is positively reinforced (through parental attention, game playing, etc.) for crying/throwing a tantrum at bedtime or when he/she awakens during the night. As stated above, many children with sleep problems may have learned to expect that their parents will respond when they cry; because of this association, they are unable to initiate sleep on their own. Thus a withdrawal of that positive reinforcement (i.e., by ignoring the child) should result in a decrease in the problem behavior. The several methods of applying extinction are outlined in the following material.

In a basic extinction program, parents are instructed to put their child to bed at a specified time and not return to the child until the next morning at a specified time. Parents are to ignore all screaming, crying, etc. When the child first cries, the parent can check to ensure the child is safe, but this checking should be done in a matter-of-fact manner, with little attention given to the child. Thereafter the parent should ignore any crying or tantrum throwing. Extinction can produce quick results (a significant decrease in crying within several days) and is generally easy for parents to understand. However, extinction can be difficult for parents to implement, because they often have a difficult time ignoring their child's crying and may end up attending to this behavior. This attention can be counterproductive, as parents may reinforce the crying, intermittently, thereby making it more difficult to extinguish this behavior. Some parents find extinction to be unacceptable and are unwilling to use such a technique (France et al., 1996; Kuhn & Weidinger, 2000; Mindell, 1999).

For parents who are unwilling to use an unmodified extinction method, or in situations in which extinction is not advised (e.g., with children who have undergone previous multiple attempts at sleep programs in the past; France et al., 1996), variations to the above program can be made. Gradual extinction programs are based on the same principle (not responding to the aversive behavior will result in a decrease in this behavior), but instead of completely ignoring the child, parents are instructed to modify how they attend to the child; generally, instead of completely ignoring their crying child, parents gradually reduce the attention they give in response to the crying.

Modified attention withdrawal is typically accomplished in one of two ways. In one method, the parent ignores the child's tantrums and crying, as above, but checks on the child at set time intervals (e.g., every 10 minutes). When the parent checks on the child, the parent should briefly comfort him/her (e.g., give the child a pat on the back, say "good-night"—no extended attention) and then leave. Typically, the time period that the parent waits before returning to comfort the child is gradually increased. For example, initially the parent may check on the child every 10 minutes, then every 15, then every 20 minutes, as the child develops better self-soothing skills (France et al., 1996; Kuhn & Weidinger, 2000; Mindell, 1999). This method may be more acceptable to parents than complete attention withdrawal, though it may have the adverse effect of prolonging the crying (particularly immediately after the parent checks on the child). It also may take more time for the crying/nighttime waking to resolve (France et al., 1996).

In another method of gradual attention withdrawal, the parent immediately responds to the child but gradually decreases the amount of time spent with the child (France et al., 1996; Kuhn & Weidinger, 2000; Mindell, 1999). For example, perhaps prior to treatment the parent was spending 30 minutes helping the child return to sleep. During treatment, initially the parent would spend 20 minutes with the child, then 15, then 10, eventually reducing this time to a brief interaction as part of the bedtime routine. Depending on how gradually the time the parent spends with the child is reduced, this program may take longer than other programs. Still, parents may find this program more acceptable because of its gradual steps and the fact that they are still spending time with their child.

Extinction also can be used with the parent present. When using this method, the parent sets up a bed for him/herself in the child's room. (It is important that this method be applied in the child's bedroom, not the parents', for obvious reasons.) If the child cries after being put in bed, the parent lays down on his/her bed and pretends to be asleep. The parent then leaves when the child falls asleep but returns and repeats this procedure if the child awakens and cries during the night. The parent continues doing this for one week and then proceeds with the complete withdrawal of attention, as outlined above. This program is most appropriate for parents who are willing to change their sleeping arrangements. It may be particularly useful for children who are accustomed to having their parents present as they fall asleep, and for children who may have some separation anxiety related to bedtime (France et al., 1996; Kuhn & Weidinger, 2000).

With any of the extinction programs, once the child is regularly sleeping through the night, the parents can stop the program. If the child does cry, the parent can briefly check on him/her. If the child has awakened because of an illness or bad dream, the parent would give attention, as appropriate; otherwise the parent's attention should be very brief. If sleep problems recur after the program has been stopped, parents should immediately reinstate it (France et al., 1996). As a supplement to the extinction procedures, parents also may want to consider using a reinforcement program for the child, in which he/she would receive a reinforcer in the morning if he/she stays in his/her bed all night and does not cry (France et al., 1996).

With all extinction programs parents should be told what to expect in terms of child behaviors. The "extinction burst" is one of the most important concepts of which parents should be aware. With all programs that incorporate ignoring, it is common for the child's behaviors to increase in duration and intensity prior to decreasing. A "spontaneous recovery" of the problem behavior after a seemingly successful intervention is also common. In this situation, the child improves initially but then reverts to exhibiting the same problem behaviors. When such a regression occurs, parents should stick with the program they are using and not return to attending, at length, to the child's crying, as this attention will only serve to delay and complicate extinction of the problem behavior (France et al., 1996).

Scheduled Wakings

Scheduled wakings also have been recommended for children who have difficulties going back to sleep after waking during the night. In order to utilize this technique, parents must first record when their child typically awakens during the night, then awaken their child 15–30 minutes prior to this time. After waking the child, the parent comforts the child, as was done when the child awoke on his/her own. Gradually the parent lengthens the time he/she waits before waking the child so that the child learns to sleep for longer periods of time. Although this treatment method may seem somewhat counterintuitive, the parent is basically shaping the child's sleep time by gradually teaching the child to sleep longer. Thus the child's sleep time gradually increases, and spontaneous wakings are eliminated (Kuhn & Weidinger, 2000; Mindell, 1999).

Bedtime Pass

Another treatment option for children who awaken and also leave the bedroom is the use of a "bedtime pass," as described by Friman et al. (1999). When using this method, the child is given a bedtime pass (created from an index card or some other form of paper) prior to going to sleep. The child is informed that he/she can use the pass for one out-of-bedroom experience per night. The child must use the pass for a specific activity (e.g., getting a drink, going to the bathroom) and must surrender the pass to his/her parents after using it. Once the child has used his/her pass, all other crying is ignored, and the straying child is immediately returned to his/her room. Although Friman et al. specified the use of only one pass, children who awaken frequently during the night may be given several passes initially and the number tapered off over time.

Arousal Disorders

Sleep terrors and sleepwalking are types of arousal disorders that may be seen in children. These disorders share similar features, including disorientation, difficulty being aroused, and lack of recall for the episode. These behaviors occur at a specific time during the sleep cycle, generally 1 to 3 hours after the onset of sleep. There appears to be a developmental progression to these disorders, in that they often disappear or significantly decrease once adolescence is reached (Anders & Eiben, 1997; Mindell, 1996). A summary of these problems and suggested intervention methods are provided below, and a handout for parents is provided in Figure 5.13.

Sleep Terrors

Sleep terrors or night terrors occur in 3–6% of children. A child having a sleep terror will awaken suddenly and scream or cry as well as manifest fear. Children are typically difficult to soothe during a sleep terror episode and may actually become more agitated when soothing attempts are made (Mindell, 1993, 1996).

Because children typically outgrow sleep terrors, and because these episodes have no negative impact on the child, there is no real treatment plan for this disorder. However, parents can make some modifications that may reduce the occurrence of sleep terrors. A lack of sleep or unusual stress can exacerbate sleep terrors (and other arousal disorders). Thus parents should ensure that their child is following a regular sleep routine and is getting an adequate amount of sleep. In addition, any unusual stressors in the child's life should be addressed, if possible. Educating parents (and the child, too) about the nature of sleep terrors also is appropriate, and parents should be assured that the sleep terrors are not a sign of an underlying psychological problem. In addition, because attempting to awaken and reassure a child having a sleep terror can result in increased agitation, parents should be instructed to avoid intervening unless the child's safety becomes an issue (Anders & Eiben, 1997; Mindell, 1996). Scheduled wakings (described above) also may help reduce episodes of sleep terrors (Mindell, 1996; Stores, 2001).

Sleep terrors should be differentiated from nightmares, which are frightening dreams that may waken the child. Nightmares typically occur during the second half of the night, and children are often able to recall the dream content. Nightmares are common in young children, with estimates of occurrence in children ages 3 to 6 ranging from 10–50%. As with the arousal disorders, nightmares tend to decrease as the child ages (Anders & Eiben, 1997; Mindell, 1996). Nightmares can be exacerbated by stress but, in general, are seen as a typical part of development (Shroeder & Gordan, 2002; Thiedke, 2001). In extreme cases, children may develop a fear or anxiety about bedtime because of nightmares. If this reaction occurs, the procedures discussed in Chapter 4 regarding the treatment of anxiety disorders should be used. For example, desensitization may be used to depotentiate the content of the child's nightmare. Obviously, if the child is having nightmares due to exposure to frightening stimuli during the day, the child's exposure to these stimuli should be reduced (Schroeder & Gordan, 2002). In general, the only "treatment" recommended for nightmares is reassurance by parents at the time of the nightmare. Recounting the nightmare may be beneficial for some children but lead to increased distress for others. Thus parents may want to ask the child if he/she would like to talk about the nightmare, but they should not pressure the child to do so (Mindell, 1996).

SLEEP TERRORS/SLEEPWALKING/NIGHTMARES: INFORMATION FOR PARENTS

Sleep Terrors

Definition: The child suddenly screams, appears fearful, and is unresponsive to parental attempts to soothe. If the child is awakened he/she may appear more agitated and disoriented. These episodes can be upsetting for parents, but the child typically returns to sleep within 5 minutes and has no memory of the incident later. Sleep terrors typically occur 1–3 hours after the child falls asleep.

What to do: Do not attempt to awaken the child—simply make sure he/she is safe. Because sleep terrors can be related to lack of sleep, make sure your child is getting an adequate amount of sleep and following an appropriate bedtime routine. Sleep terrors also may occur more in times of stress so stressors should be identified and reduced, if possible.

Sleepwalking

Definition: The child actually gets out of bed and walks around the house. This behavior typically occurs 1–3 hours after the child falls asleep.

What to do: As with sleep terrors, do not attempt to awaken your child—simply lead him/her back to bed in a calm manner. Because sleepwalking can be dangerous for the child, prevention of injury is essential. Parents should ensure that windows and doors are shut and locked. If the child's bedroom is not on the first floor, install a gate at the top of the stairs. Parents also may consider rigging some type of alarm system that will notify them when their child is out of his/her room. Bells, tin cans, or some other noise-making device may be tied to the child's door so that when it is opened, the parents are awakened. As with sleep terrors, it is important that the child is getting enough sleep and that stress is reduced, if possible.

Nightmares

Definition: Nightmares are frightening dreams that may awaken the child and typically occur in the second half of the night. The child likely will remember these dreams in the morning.

What to do: Provide comfort to the child at the time the nightmare occurs. Give the child an opportunity to talk about the nightmare but do not pressure him/her to do so.

FIGURE 5.13. Sleep terrors/sleepwalking/nightmares: information for parents. From Gretchen A. Gimpel and Melissa L. Holland (2003). Copyright by The Guilford Press. Permission to photocopy this figure is granted to purchasers of this book for personal use only (see copyright page for details).

Sleepwalking

Sleepwalking can involve limited movement to walks around the house. Because of the potential for harm when a child sleepwalks, parents should attempt to minimize unsafe situations. For example, outside doors as well as windows should be shut and locked, and the child's bedroom should be on the first floor, if possible. In addition, parents may want to consider installing some type of mechanism that will alert them to when their child is up. For example, bells may be attached to the child's door. When parents interact with their sleepwalking child, they should not yell at or shake the child but gradually lead him/her back to the bedroom. Scheduled wakings (discussed above) also may be used to attempt to reduce the incidence of sleepwalking (Mindell, 1996; Thiedke, 2001).

CHAPTER SUMMARY

This chapter provided a review of treatments for common, everyday problems frequently exhibited by young children. Although many parents do not initially consult with mental health professionals regarding these problems, mental health professionals trained in behavioral interventions are excellent resources for parents of children having problems with toileting, feeding, or sleeping. The empirically supported interventions for these disorders are all based on behavioral methods of reinforcing appropriate behaviors (e.g., attending to appropriate eating behaviors, giving praise and tangible reinforcers for having a bowel movement in the toilet) and ignoring or providing a mildly aversive consequence for inappropriate behaviors (e.g., ignoring crying at bedtime, using time-out for inappropriate eating behaviors). Although the problems discussed in this chapter are often not indicative of later psychopathology, providing treatment can significantly reduce problematic parent–child interactions and potentially preclude stressful social experiences for the child.

6

Working with Young Children Who Have Been Abused

It is widely recognized that child abuse can have multiple adverse effects on children who have been abused, the families of these children, and society as a whole. Physical abuse, sexual abuse, emotional abuse, and neglect all can significantly impact a child's physical and psychological well-being and disrupt normal childhood development. The longstanding psychological effects of child abuse are well documented (Briere, 1992), including the increased potential that an abused child will become an abuser as an adult. Within the United States alone, in 1995, there were approximately 1 million substantiated reports of child maltreatment and 1,000 child deaths due to child neglect or abuse (U.S. Department of Health and Human Services, 1997). This chapter provides an overview of the definitions and effects of abuse, discusses interventions that can be used for young children who have been abused, and summarizes prevention methods for parents, teachers, and professionals working with the preschool and kindergarten population.

OVERVIEW OF PHYSICAL, SEXUAL, AND EMOTIONAL ABUSE AND NEGLECT

States have somewhat differing definitions of what constitutes abuse and neglect of children. Professionals working with children should become familiar with their state's specific definitions and regulations regarding abuse. This section provides an overview of broad definitions for each area.

Broadly defined, *physical abuse* is the infliction of injury, other than by accidental means, on a child by another person. Hitting, biting, kicking, beating, shoving, burning, pulling out hair, or other nonaccidental methods of causing bodily harm to a child would be covered under this definition.

Sexual abuse of a child usually refers to sexual assault or exploitation of a minor by an adult, or between two children when one of the children is significantly older or there is a significant power differential between the children (e.g., one child is developmentally delayed) or when coercion is used. Often included in this definition is touching of the breasts, genitals, or buttocks of a child, penetration of the anus or vagina with an object, fellatio, cunnilingus, or the prostitution, exploitation, or involvement of the child in pornography.

Neglect is often defined as the failure of a person having the care or custody of a child to provide adequate care and protection for the child. Neglect may involve failure to provide sufficient food, shelter, medical care, clothing, or supervision to a child. Educational neglect (e.g., not ensuring school attendance/depriving the child of a legally mandated education) may fall under this category.

Psychological or emotional abuse occurs when an adult conveys to a child that the child is endangered, unsafe, worthless, unwanted, or damaged; it may include verbal threats, terrorization, isolation, or frequent berating of a child by the adult. This type of abuse is not covered by mandated reporting laws in all states.

Generally, a report of abuse to the appropriate child protective agency is legally required by mental health clinicians, teachers, and other professionals, if there is a reasonable suspicion that abuse has occurred. In most states there is a strong immunity against liability for the reporter if the report of abuse is made in "good faith." Failure of a professional to report suspected abuse could result in various actions, such as fines, revocation of licenses, and/or incarceration. Again, the professional should review the relevant child-abuse reporting laws in his/her state to determine the specifics of when and how to make a report.

Additionally, the clinician who works with children should be aware of any relevant cultural practices/approaches to disciplining children. Different cultures have differing parenting practices; terminology surrounding those practices and the cultural heritage and religious beliefs of the family should be explored and taken into consideration when working with the child (American Academy of Child and Adolescent Psychiatry, 1997b). For example, if a child reports that he/she is "whooped" at home, try to determine whether this means (1) spanked with an open hand occasionally when misbehaving, (2) hit with a closed fist, (3) hit with an object, or (4) hit on different parts of the body. It is important to reiterate, though, that if abuse or neglect is suspected, a child-abuse report is mandated, regardless of the mitigating circumstances surrounding the event. It is not the clinician's duty to make sense of the surrounding circumstances; it is the clinician's duty to report any suspected abuse so that the appropriate authorities can investigate the situation.

Often with preschool- and kindergarten-age children the best "window" into the child's world is through observing the child's behaviors. Children rarely verbally report abuse, particularly if the perpetrator is the child's parent. However, if a child does verbalize allegations, it is essential to make a child-abuse report.

EFFECTS OF CHILD ABUSE

As mentioned previously, there are a number of different effects that abuse and neglect can have on young children. This section reviews the more salient ones. A handout summarizing some of the symptoms to look for is provided in Figure 6.1. However, do not assume that abuse has taken place solely because some of these behaviors are present; these problems are not unique to children who have been abused. At the same time, be aware that abuse may be an issue if a child is exhibiting several of these symptoms.

Physical Effects

The most obvious signs of abuse and neglect are the physical signs and effects. In the case of physical abuse, bruises, fractures, lacerations, burns, facial or head injuries, or other physical injuries that cannot be explained, or for which improbable explanations are given, are commonly seen. For a child suffering from sexual abuse, bruising or tearing around the genital or anal area, visible lesions about the mouth or genitals, painful urination or defecation, rectal or vaginal pain or bleeding, or the complaint of lower abdominal pain may be present. For a child who has been neglected, failure to thrive (e.g., passivity, apathy toward environment, lack of weight gain), or failure to make expected weight gains, may be seen. Other physical indicators of neglect include unkempt appearance, dirty clothing or hair, offensive body odor, malnutrition, frequent illness, poor oral hygiene, poor muscle tone, or unattended medical conditions, such as infections of the skin. Though there are no physical signs of emotional abuse, this type of abuse often co-occurs with physical or sexual abuse or neglect.

Psychological Effects

The psychological and emotional effects of abuse are often more difficult to detect than the physical effects. Unfortunately, the psychological effects also often cause more longstanding difficulties for the child and may lead to mental health problems well into adulthood (Briere, 1992). Therefore, the detection and treatment of these effects are imperative. Children who have been abused can exhibit a wide array of psychological difficulties, and there is no set pattern of symptoms that is typical of all children who have been abused. Young children who have been physically abused frequently exhibit problems with attachment and engage in aggressive behaviors. In addition, they may be withdrawn or anxious. Children who have been sexually abused may have some of the same symptoms (e.g., behavior problems, anxiety) in addition to sexual acting-out behavior or oversexualized behavior—one of the symptoms unique to sexual abuse (Becker & Bonner, 1998; State of California Department of Social Services, 1997). Young children who have been sexually abused may engage in inappropriate levels of sexual behavior (e.g., excessive masturbation), may know sexual terms most children their age do not, or otherwise exhibit high levels of sexualized behaviors.

Although the majority of abused children will experience some psychological distress, not all children who have been abused will have psychological symptoms. In some children who are initially asymptomatic, effects will be noted later (a phenomenon known as the "sleeper effect"), whereas psychological effects may never be noted in other children. Children who never show effects may have a number of resiliency factors (e.g., supportive family members, good social skills), and/or the abuse may not have been traumatic enough to the child to produce harmful psychological effects (Saywitz, Mannarino, Berliner, & Cohen, 2000).

SIGNS AND SYMPTOMS OF ABUSE

There is no single set of symptoms associated with child abuse. Different children react differently to being abused. However, some symptoms have been found to be consistently related to child abuse and neglect. This list is not meant to be exhaustive, and many of these behaviors may overlap across different forms of abuse. Obviously, just because a child is exhibiting one (or more) of these behaviors does not mean the child was abused or neglected. Instead these behaviors are to be considered "red flags" that there could be a potential problem that may require some form of intervention.

Physical Effects of Abuse

Physical abuse
- Bruises, fractures, lacerations, burns, facial or head injuries, or other physical injuries that cannot be explained or for which improbable explanations are given

Sexual abuse
- Bruising or tearing around the genital or anal area, visible lesions about the mouth or genitals, painful urination or defecation, rectal or vaginal pain or bleeding, and the complaint of lower abdominal pain

Neglect
- Failure to thrive (e.g., passivity, apathy toward environment, lack of weight gain) or failure to make expected weight gains, unkempt appearance, dirty clothing or hair, offensive body odor, malnutrition, frequent illness, poor oral hygiene, poor muscle tone, or unattended medical conditions such as infections of the skin

Psychological Effects of Abuse

Physical abuse
- Aggressive, oppositional, or destructive behavior
- Self-destructiveness, head banging, suicidality
- Use of foul language/verbally abusive
- Extreme fear/withdrawn or isolative behaviors
- Frequent tantrums/out-of-control behaviors
- Insecure attachments with caregivers
- Frequently violent or destructive play themes
- Animal abuse

Sexual Abuse
- Sexualized behaviors or talk
- Frequent/inappropriate masturbation
- Aggressiveness/hostility
- Fearful or isolative behaviors
- Insecure attachments with caregivers
- Self-destructive behaviors
- Sexualized play themes

(continued)

FIGURE 6.1. Signs and symptoms of abuse. From Gretchen A. Gimpel and Melissa L. Holland (2003). Copyright by The Guilford Press. Permission to photocopy this figure is granted to purchasers of this book for personal use only (see copyright page for details).

Neglect
- Depression/passivity
- Withdrawn/isolative behaviors
- Overly attached to outsiders/clingy
- Delayed cognitive or speech skills

Emotional Abuse
- Hostile, aggressive, or verbally abusive to others
- Depression/lack of self-esteem
- Overly seeking of others' approval
- Fear of rejection/unable to make choices or decisions

In addition to the behavioral indicators of abuse, children who have been victims of abuse or neglect may develop trauma-specific disorders. It is becoming increasingly recognized that young children exposed to trauma may develop posttraumatic stress disorder (PTSD) (Kaufman & Henrich, 2000; Scheeringa & Gaensbauer, 2000). It is estimated that approximately 50% of children who have been sexually abused will exhibit symptoms of PTSD (Saywitz et al., 2000). Reactive attachment disorder, which involves a prominent disturbance in a young child's social relatedness, evident early in life in association with pathogenic care, also may develop after ongoing abuse or severe neglect (Kaufman & Henrich, 2000).

INTERVENTIONS FOR YOUNG CHILDREN WHO HAVE BEEN ABUSED

Preschool and kindergarten children who have been traumatized present unique challenges to the professionals working with them. First and foremost, it is often difficult for the child to express in words exactly what happened to him/her or to be able to verbally process feelings or thoughts associated with the abuse. As discussed in Chapter 2, interviewing young children, though important, can be difficult and fraught with problems. Preschoolers' memories may be unreliable because they do not possess as many schemas for organizing and retrieving specific memories as do older children. Therefore, memories may be distorted to conform to an existing schema (Shelby, 2000). For example, a child may report that the abuser was a "monster" because he/she does not have a preexisting schema for a child molester. The professional working with the child should be aware of these embellishments in the memories of the young child but not dismiss the child simply because his/her report does not make logical sense.

Because there are significant variations in the familial, environmental, cultural, developmental, and clinical characteristics of abuse, it is unlikely that any one intervention would be appropriate for all victims (Kaufman & Henrich, 2000). Each child's circumstances and situation must be considered individually, along with the child's presenting symptoms. Because the symptoms that may be exhibited by children who have been abused vary so much, as discussed above, it is important that the clinician conduct a thorough assessment of the child and his/her family in order to target the areas in which the child is having the most difficulty.

First and foremost, the initial step in the treatment of child abuse is to ensure the current and continued safety of child. This *safety* refers to both the physical safety of the child in his/her environment and the safety the child feels in the therapeutic setting (Scheeringa & Gaensbauer, 2000). As discussed earlier, if abuse is suspected or reported by the child or caregiver, the professional working with the child has an obligation to report the abuse to the child protective authorities. Ongoing monitoring of the situation and consultation with the appropriate child protective agency personnel following the report are necessary in determining if the child continues to be exposed to an abusive situation. For example, does the child still live with, or have contact with, the abuser? If so, is the abuse continuing? If further abuse is suspected, the clinician must take action to ensure that the child is protected. Typically, the clinician would file another child-abuse report. If possible, when such a report is made, the caregivers should be informed and the clinician should discuss with them the steps they need to take to ensure the safety of the child. Obviously the specific steps to be taken would depend on the child's situation. Child protective agencies normally offer numerous services geared toward ensuring the child's safety. However, the report should be made without the knowledge of the caregivers if informing them is likely to injure the child further. The best interests of the child, in accordance with local and state laws and regulations, should always be the guiding principle for what action to take. However, clinicians should make sure they do not fall into the trap of not reporting suspected abuse because they believe it is better for the child that a report not be made (e.g., they are concerned that the family will terminate ongoing therapy services if they know a report has been made). Collaboration between protective services, social workers, the therapist, and the school may be both helpful and necessary in the effective treatment of the child. It is recommended that the child who has been abused receive services from a mental health professional trained in working with abused children.

Treatment of the family system is often crucial in cases of child abuse. Family therapy, parent therapy, or parent training may be appropriate in many cases, regardless of who perpetrated the abuse. Research has suggested that parent intervention is a critical component in the treatment of children who have been sexually abused (Deblinger, McLeer, & Henry, 1990). Many parents find it useful to be able to have access to a forum in which they can discuss their fears and concerns, particularly if the perpetrator was another family member or family friend. If the parent was the abuser, seminars in anger management and effective parenting techniques would be important in helping the parent develop effective and acceptable means of parenting and disciplinary practices, especially if the abuse was physical in nature. Often siblings are not fully informed of the circumstances or issues surrounding the abuse, though the abuse likely impacts them either directly or indirectly, and family sessions can be one way to include the siblings (Glaser, 1991). If the child is removed from the home, the therapist should make every effort to continue the individual work with the child, thereby providing both consistency and stability. Foster care and adoptive families that take in abused children will need information about working with these children, including how to manage difficult behaviors, sexual issues that may arise, and determining the place of the biological family in the children's lives (Glaser, 1991). Because a stable home environment can facilitate the healing process, it is recommended that children who have experienced abuse or neglect not be subjected to continually changing living arrangements and caregivers (Mayhall & Norgard, 1983).

Once the child's physical safety is established, the therapeutic work should focus on helping him/her feel psychologically safe. The therapy room should be perceived as a warm, safe place, with minimal distractions and a nurturing atmosphere. The establishment of rapport between the therapist and child, of course, is key. Therapists should remain nondirective (particularly initially) and child-focused. Clinicians who ask the child detailed, probing questions about the abuse during the initial sessions may seem threatening to the child, potentially causing the child to feel unsafe and possibly further traumatizing him/her. Extra support measures during the therapy may be necessary, such as increased sessions during the week, check-in phone calls with the family between sessions, or, if available, having a mentor or case manager visit the child in the home to provide support to both the child and the family.

Some structure should be introduced in the first sessions via reviewing the role of the therapist, the purpose of therapy, and the "rules" of the playroom. An example of this initial presentation by the therapist follows.

> "My name is Kelly. I am someone children come and play with or talk to about things that are bothering them. Sometimes in here we will talk about things, sometimes we will play. You can play with whatever you want to in here. We will meet each week for about 45 minutes. There are only three rules in here. The first rule is that you cannot hurt yourself, the second rule is that you cannot hurt me, and the third rule is that you cannot hurt the toys. Also, all of the toys stay here in this room; you cannot take toys home with you. Other than that, we can do what you would like in here.
>
> Everything that you do in here and talk about in here will stay between you and me. I won't tell anyone about it, unless you are going to hurt yourself or hurt someone else, or if someone else is hurting you. If one of those things is happening, I will have to tell someone to make sure that you are safe. We can talk about it if any of those things come up. Do you have any questions about anything I just said?"

Obviously this is a lot for a young child to take in at the first session. Reviewing the rules, or any other aspect of the therapy, likely will be necessary during future sessions.

Young children, in particular, may regress to a previously safe developmental level, and behaviors such as thumbsucking, baby talk, and wetting may occur. Toys younger than the child's developmental level should be available in case the child prefers to revert to a safer time in his/her life. Common toys used for young children who have been abused include (but are not limited to) large pillows and blankets, baby bottles, sand trays, puppets, doll families and dollhouses, crayons/paints and paper, dinosaurs and animal figures, play food and dishes, dress-up clothes, and baby dolls. Play should be allowed to occur freely and at any developmental level the child wishes to function at during the session. Observation and description, including interpretation of the child's activities, are often useful if the child will allow it. Sometimes even following of the child's activities verbally may prove to be too much; instead, the child may need an adult simply to be present in the room, observing his/her play. Below is an example of a therapist verbally tracking the play of a 5-year-old child who was sexually molested by his stepfather:

CHILD: (*Engages in doll play involving an adult male doll and a child doll, with the child doll hitting the adult male doll.*)

THERAPIST: That little boy is feeling angry at that man. He wants to hurt him.

CHILD: (*Continues in the play, intensifying the hitting of the adult male doll.*)

THERAPIST: That little boy wants that man to know how mad he is at him.

CHILD: (*Continues in the play, then throws the dolls into the dollhouse. Walks over to the pillows and blankets and lies down.*)

THERAPIST: You are feeling a little tired after feeling so many feelings. You are resting now.

As shown in this example, the therapist verbally follows the actions the child is making during his play. This nondirective approach allows the child to lead the session and feel heard by the therapist; the therapist, in turn, avoids any leading or directive questions or interpretations (Axeline, 1969). Invasiveness by the therapist can prove to be retraumatizing to the abused child, further violating already violated boundaries and limits. Gil (1991) has written about nonintrusive therapy, suggesting that "because physical and sexual abuse are intrusive acts, the clinician's interventions should be nonintrusive, allowing the child ample physical and emotional space" (p. 59).

Evident in the previous example is the child's reenactment of some of the trauma through the doll play. Selecting the two figures and expressing anger and violence allow the child to process difficult feelings around the abuse without confronting these overwhelming feelings more directly. Repetition in the play helps the child to reenact the trauma via therapeutic and developmentally appropriate means while working through it. This process is consistent with that undergone by the traumatized adult who, in therapy, retells his/her story, again and again, in order to make meaning of, and eventually "let go" of, the stressful event. Aggressive and attacking behaviors exhibited by the abused child in therapy, though often disturbing to teachers and new clinicians, can offer a way for the child to replace feelings of fear with feelings of control, safety, and power (Gil, 1991). Toward the end of successful therapy, these children usually begin to exhibit healthier and more developmentally appropriate play, and they are able to discontinue the repetitive play reenacting the trauma.

Although nondirective, supportive interventions have a lengthy history in the treatment of abused children, cognitive-behavioral therapy (CBT) interventions are increasingly being used to treat children (and their families) who have been abused. Such treatments make use of a variety of techniques to target the specific symptoms exhibited by the child. For example, for a child with symptoms of anxiety, relaxation training and systematic desensitization (as outlined in Chapter 4) may be useful treatments. In general, the research literature is supportive of the use of CBT techniques with children who have been abused; however, more research with rigorous methodology is needed in this area (Saywitz et al., 2000). CBT techniques are discussed in more detail in the section on post-traumatic stress disorder.

Therapists, teachers, and other professionals working with the children who have been abused should be aware of the emotional impact this type of work may have on them and take steps to ensure their own emotional well being as well as prevent burnout (Glaser, 1991). Supportive measures for professionals include attending structured or unstructured consultation groups focused on abuse cases, discussing with other professionals personal feelings that come up while working with abused children, and/or engaging in therapy to address difficult thoughts and feelings that may arise. Professionals should always be aware of and monitor their feelings and take steps necessary to take care of themselves during this difficult work.

POSTTRAUMATIC STRESS DISORDER

Posttraumatic stress disorder (PTSD), as reviewed in Chapter 4, is an anxiety disorder that emerges when a child has been exposed to some form of trauma. Not every child exposed to a traumatic event will develop PTSD symptoms; however, as noted, it is common for children to develop PTSD symptoms (including reexperiencing the trauma, avoiding the stimuli associated with the trauma, and unpleasant symptoms of increased arousal; American Psychiatric Association, 1994) following abuse as well as following other traumatic events.

The reexperiencing of the trauma occurs in different ways for different children, though most often the trauma is "played out" through the use of toys in the case of young children. A child who has experienced abuse, for example, may play out the abuse with dolls, reenacting the experience over and over again (as in the example provided previously). A child who has experienced a natural disaster may draw the chaos repeatedly with crayons or may replay the experience using toys that resemble objects or structures present during the disaster (Scheeringa & Gaensbauer, 2000).

In addition to anxiety and the reliving of the trauma, young children with PTSD also often exhibit depressive symptoms, behavioral problems, anger, withdrawal from social contact, and school-related difficulties (such as not progressing with learned concepts or acting out). For some children, these symptoms are the first indication that they are having problems.

The most common forms of trauma to which young children are exposed include abuse and neglect, witnessing domestic violence, witnessing community violence, natural disasters, accidents, and painful medical procedures (Scheeringa & Gaensbauer, 2000). It is difficult to prevent PTSD symptoms, due to the typically uncontrollable/unpredictable nature of these types of stressors. Different children respond differently to stressors as a result of past learning, physiological makeup, social supports available, and coping strategies. A child who has been exposed to a traumatic stimulus and evidences symptoms of PTSD should receive immediate intervention to decrease the severity of the symptoms. Left untreated, PTSD can have an impact upon subsequent social and psychological maturation, potentially leading to atypical and dysfunctional development (Briere, 1992).

Treatment of PTSD in Young Children

As discussed regarding abuse, the initial step in the treatment of PTSD is to ensure the safety of the child and to make certain that the child is no longer being exposed to the traumatic circumstances. It is almost impossible to attempt to treat a child for trauma when he/she continues to be traumatized in his/her environment. Obviously, psychological safety (discussed previously) also is important.

As with treatments for the variety of symptoms associated with abuse, CBT has the most empirical support for addressing symptoms of PTSD in children. Many CBT programs have treatment components for both the child and the parent. With young children, in particular, this combined treatment approach likely will be the most efficacious.

Parents may be involved in interventions in several ways. Many parents will need some basic information regarding childhood PTSD, including the diagnostic criteria and childhood presentation of the disorder as well as a description of the course of treatment. It also may be helpful to give parents information about child sexual abuse, normal sexuality, and ways in which they can help their child feel personally safe. In addition to education, parents of abused children often need psychological assistance themselves, as they frequently experience some emotional distress due to their child's abuse. Parents may benefit from specific interventions directed to them, such as cognitive strategies to decrease self-blame and exposure techniques related to their thoughts and feelings about their child's abuse (Cohen, Mannarino, Berliner, & Deblinger, 2000; Olafson & Boat, 2000). Parent training (as discussed in Chapter 3) also may be part of a CBT program to help parents address aggressive, acting-out behaviors exhibited by their child as well as reinforce appropriate behaviors and provide positive, child-directed time at home (King et al., 2000). Because harsh discipline or punishment can worsen a traumatized child's feelings of low self-esteem and insecurity, disciplinary methods should be executed in a patient and nonpunitive manner (Scheeringa & Gaensbauer, 2000). Lastly, increasing the structure in home and school activities can help reduce the child's anxiety.

Child-directed components that may be part of a CBT intervention package include psychoeducation, coping skills training, social skills training, and gradual exposure. Psychoeducation often includes age-appropriate information on sexuality and sexual abuse as well as personal safety skills to assist children with avoiding (to the extent possible) future abuse incidents. Coping skills training includes interventions that assist children in dealing with the distressing, dysfunctional thoughts related to the abuse. Techniques used may include relaxation training (as discussed in Chapter 4) as well as cognitive coping skills similar to those used with children who have depression or anxiety disorders. These techniques, which have been used with some success with children with PTSD, include replacing negative, maladaptive thoughts with more positive, coping thoughts, and addressing self-blame and cognitive distortions (Cohen et al., 2000; King et al., 2000). Relaxation techniques can be useful in decreasing any physical symptoms of arousal the child continues to experience. Because children often evidence increased aggressive behaviors and/or problematic social behaviors following instances of abuse, some training in social skills/social problem solving (discussed in Chapter 3) may be beneficial (King et al., 2000).

Gradual exposure, a key component in CBT interventions for PTSD, is considered by many to be the most important part of a successful treatment program for this disorder. The same basic format discussed in Chapter 4 for systematic desensitization is used with gradual exposure. Children construct an anxiety hierarchy composed of aspects of the abuse or the abuser with items that are less anxiety provoking (e.g., interactions with the abuser at times he/she was not abusing the child) at the bottom, and items that are extremely anxiety-provoking (e.g., specifics about the abuse event) at the top. The clinician gradually takes the child through the hierarchy of items. Exposure to the items may be done via talking about them, drawing, story telling, playing, or any other method that is appropriate for the child's age and developmental level. As part of the gradual exposure, relaxation training and positive self-talk may be used as mechanisms for coping with the anxiety (King et al., 2000).

Young children who are still in the grip of reliving their trauma also often have nightmares and difficulties sleeping and eating. The content of the child's dreams may not be recognizable to the child, except for the fact that the dream was anxiety provoking. Reading soothing bedtime stories, engaging in regular bedtime and mealtime routines, and frequent comforting and reassurance by the parent are recommended. Communication between the child's clinician and parents is important to monitor and treat these related symptoms.

PREVENTION METHODS FOR PARENTS AND TEACHERS

Because child abuse and neglect can have long-term negative consequences, considerable effort has been directed toward its prevention. Ideally, prevention measures should be founded on an understanding of the risk factors that can lead to child abuse and neglect and services rendered before the abuse begins. Common risk factors for abuse and neglect are reviewed here, along with services to aid the family. This approach would be considered one of "primary prevention." "Secondary prevention" involves the early identification and treatment of child abuse and neglect. "Tertiary prevention" is considered rehabilitative: The abuse has occurred for an extended period of time, and intervention is necessary to change set family patterns. Though secondary and tertiary measures constitute treatments, they also are preventive if they are successful at thwarting further abuse and neglect within the family system or further problems associated with the abuse and neglect (Mayhall & Norgard, 1983). Because interventions have been discussed earlier in this chapter, this section focuses primarily on primary prevention methods.

Primary prevention—that is, determining risk factors and intervening before any abuse has occurred—is often conducted by teachers, daycare providers, and other professionals who work closely with the young child on a daily basis and have the opportunity to make frequent observations. Risk factors often co-occur and are cumulative; no single risk factor is indicative of a potentially abusive situation, though several risk factors could render the family more vulnerable to abusive events. Common risk factors include premature birth of the child, depressive symptoms and anxiety in the mother, single parent situations, families experiencing divorce or those with significant marital discord, coercive discipline, and poverty and associated factors (such as low education levels, substance use, criminal activity, and crowded conditions) (Beckwith, 2000).

If several of these risk factors are present, professionals could intervene via connecting the parents or family with appropriate social services. For example, in the case of the use of coercive discipline, the parent could (1) be given resources (such as handouts and books) for positive parenting skills, or (2) encouraged to attend classes in effective disciplinary tactics for young children. In many situations, it also is appropriate to provide parents with individual parent training (as discussed in Chapter 3) to help them break the coercive parenting cycle. Parents who appear to have a mental health need should be encouraged to seek individual treatment. Families going through a difficult divorce situation or experiencing frequent marital discord should be given resources for martial or family therapy services or links with legal services to aid in the separation process. Social services can offer assistance to families experiencing financial hardship and other stressors related to financially impoverished situations, such as the need for food, jobs, and appropriate housing.

Helping families with risk factors make positive connections with other people may also reduce the risk of child abuse and neglect (Mayhall & Norgard, 1983). Connections provide outlets for frustrations and offer resources and alternative perspectives during stressful times. Connection also keeps families from feeling isolated. Anyone can make a connection with a family in need—teachers, social workers, daycare providers, friends, physicians and nurses, therapists, and school psychologists. Individuals who have made a connection with a family could then suggest further resources, such as becoming involved in a service or program that could address the family's specific needs.

Preventive factors—conditions that increase resiliency and resistance to conditions of adversity—can be identified and reinforced. Such factors may be child-related, such as innate intelligence or talents, or parent-related, such as having appropriate disciplinary skills or adequate social support (Beckwith, 2000). Preventive factors, just like risk factors, are cumulative; the more coping skills and resiliency the family has, the less likely it is that the family will engage in abuse. Helping the family to draw on their resiliency and positive coping styles during times of crisis can thwart the occurrence of abuse.

Many preventive resources already exist in communities to aid families at risk for abuse and neglect. Obviously the type of resource that would be most beneficial to a particular family would depend on that family's specific needs. The following is a list of resources available in many areas; in addition, the professional should familiarize him/herself with the specific resources available in the area in which the family resides.

- Parents Anonymous
- National Center for Child Abuse and Neglect
- Alcoholics/Narcotics Anonymous
- Child Protective Services
- Social services (City/County/State)
- Head Start
- Crisis nurseries and short-term emergency child placements
- Emergency housing shelters and services
- County mental health services
- Child development centers
- Various parenting or crisis hotlines
- School psychologists or counselors

Other recommended resources include those provided by the family's church or synagogue, such as counseling groups, food, and financial assistance; those offered by local universities and law schools, such as low- to no-cost counseling services, medical services (when a training hospital is affiliated) and legal advice; and services offered to the pubic by local media, such as food or clothing drives and other programs.

Other methods of prevention are directed more specifically at the child. For example, some Head Start programs use a prevention program for child sexual abuse, in which the child watches a video on good and bad forms of touching, then discusses the video and what action to take (e.g., say "no," leave, and tell a trusted adult about it) if anyone touches them in a private way. This type of prevention, using videos and/or books, also could be taught in daycares, preschools, the therapy setting, or the home.

Obviously not all programs and services will benefit all families, in part due to the heterogeneity of children and parents within a risk group. Prevention programs are most effective when they are based on prior knowledge of a child's and family's risk factors (Beckwith, 2000).

CHAPTER SUMMARY

Unfortunately, child abuse is all too prevalent in our society today. Young children, in particular, are at risk for physical and sexual abuse. Prevention of abuse is obviously the most desirable "intervention" for this problem; however, even with increased prevention efforts, abuse continues to occur. This chapter has provided a summary of interventions that may be put in place for children who have experienced abuse (or some other traumatic event) and their families. Although there is less research on effective intervention techniques for abuse and neglect than some of the other problems covered in this book, the most promising methods of treatment combine supportive therapy techniques with behavioral/cognitive-behavioral interventions, such as parenting training for parents who are abusive, and gradual exposure for children who are experiencing PTSD symptoms.

References

Achenbach, T. M. (1991a). *Manual for the Child Behavior Checklist and 1991 profile.* Burlington, VT: University of Vermont.

Achenbach, T. M. (1991b). *Manual for the Teacher's Report Form and 1991 profile.* Burlington, VT: University of Vermont.

Achenbach, T. M. (1992). *Manual for the Child Behavior Checklist/2–3 and 1992 profile.* Burlington, VT: University of Vermont.

Achenbach, T. M. (1997). *Guide for the Caregiver–Teacher Report Form for ages 2–5.* Burlington, VT: University of Vermont.

Achenbach, T. M., & Rescorla, L. A. (2000). *Manual for ASEBA Preschool Forms and Profiles.* Burlington, VT: University of Vermont.

Achenbach, T. M., & Rescorla, L. A. (2001). *Manual for ASEBA School-Age Forms and Profiles.* Burlington, VT: University of Vermont.

Albano, A. M., Chorpita, B. F., & Barlow, D. H. (2003). Childhood anxiety disorders. In E. J. Mash & R. A. Barkley (Eds.), *Child psychopathology* (2nd ed., pp. 279–329). New York: Guilford Press.

American Academy of Child and Adolescent Psychiatry. (1997a). Practice parameters for the assessment and treatment of children and adolescents with anxiety disorders. *Journal of the American Academy of Child and Adolescent Psychiatry, 36,* 69S–84S.

American Academy of Child and Adolescent Psychiatry. (1997b). Practice parameters for the psychiatric assessment of children and adolescents. *Journal of the American Academy of Child and Adolescent Psychiatry, 36,* 4S–20S.

American Academy of Child and Adolescent Psychiatry. (1998). Practice parameters for the assessment and treatment of children and adolescents with depressive disorders. *Journal of the American Academy of Child and Adolescent Psychiatry, 36,* 63S–83S.

American Academy of Child and Adolescent Psychiatry. (1999). Practice parameters for the assessment and treatment of children, adolescents, and adults with autism and other pervasive developmental disorders. *Journal of the American Academy of Child and Adolescent Psychiatry, 38,* 32S–54S.

American Psychiatric Association. (1994). *Diagnostic and statistical manual of mental disorders* (4th ed.). Washington, DC: Author.

Anastasi, A. (1997). *Psychological testing* (7th ed.). Upper Saddle River, NJ: Prentice Hall.

Anders, T. F., & Eiben, L. A. (1997). Pediatric sleep disorders: A review of the past 10 years. *Journal of the American Academy of Child and Adolescent Psychiatry, 36,* 9–20.

Axline, V. M. (1969). *Play therapy* (2nd ed.). New York: Ballantine Books.

Azrin, N. H., & Foxx, R. M. (1974). *Toilet training in less than a day.* New York: Simon & Schuster.

Babbitt, R. L., Hoch, T. A., Coe, D. A., Cataldo, M. F., Kelly, K. J., Stackhouse, C., & Perman, J. A. (1994). Behavioral assessment and treatment of pediatric feeding disorders. *Developmental and Behavioral Pediatrics, 15,* 278–291.

Baker, B. L., & Heller, T. L. (1996). Preschool children with externalizing behaviors: Experience of fathers and mothers. *Journal of Abnormal Child Psychology, 24,* 513–532.

Barkley, R. A. (1997). *Defiant children: A clinician's manual for assessment and parent training* (2nd ed.). New York: Guilford Press.

Barkley, R. A. (1998). *Attention-deficit hyperactivity disorder: A handbook for diagnosis and treatment* (2nd ed.). New York: Guilford Press.

Barkley, R. A., Shelton, T. L., Crosswait, C., Moorhouse, M., Fletcher, K., Barrett, S., Jenkins, L., & Metevia, L. (2000). Multi-method psych-educational intervention for preschool children with disruptive behavior: Preliminary results at post-treatment. *Journal of Child Psychology and Psychiatry and Allied Disciplines, 41,* 319–332.

Barrios, B. A., & O'Dell, S. L. (1998). Fears and anxieties. In E. J. Mash & R. A. Barkley (Eds.), *Treatment of childhood disorders* (2nd ed., pp. 249–337). New York: Guilford Press.

Barrish, H. H., Saunders, M., & Wolf, M. M. (1969). Good behavior game: Effects of individual contingencies for group consequences on disruptive classroom behavior. *Journal of Applied Behavior Analysis, 2,* 119–124.

Becker, J. V., & Bonner, B. (1998). Sexual and other abuse of children. In R. J. Morris & T. R. Kratochwill (Eds.), *The practice of child therapy* (3rd ed., pp. 367–389). Boston: Allyn & Bacon.

Beckwith, L. (2000). Prevention science and prevention programs. In C. H. Zeanah (Ed.), *Handbook of infant mental health* (2nd ed., pp. 439–456). New York: Guilford Press.

Bell, K. E., & Stein, D. M. (1992). Behavioral treatment for pica: A review of empirical studies. *International Journal of Eating Disorders, 11,* 377–389.

Benham, A. L. (2000). The observation and assessment of young children including use of the infant–toddler mental status exam. In C. H. Zeanah (Ed.), *Handbook of infant mental health* (2nd ed., pp. 249–265). New York: Guilford Press.

Bernstein, G. A., Borchardt, C., & Perwien, A. (1996). Anxiety disorders in children and adolescents: A review of the past 10 years. *Journal of the American Academy of Child and Adolescent Psychiatry, 35,* 1110–1119.

Biederman, J., Rosenbaum, J. F., Chaloff, J., & Kagan, J. (1995). Behavioral inhibition as a risk factor for anxiety disorders. In J. S. March (Ed.), *Anxiety disorders in children and adolescents* (pp. 61–81). New York: Guilford Press.

Birmaher, B., Ryan, N. D., Williamson, D. E., Brent, D. A., Kaufman, J., Dahl, R., Perel, J., & Nelson, B. (1996). Childhood and adolescent depression: A review of the past 10 years. Part I. *Journal of the American Academy of Child and Adolescent Psychiatry, 35,* 1427–1439.

Blondis, T. A., Snow, J. H., Stein, M., & Roizen, N. J. (1991). Appropriate use of measures of attention and activity for the diagnosis and management of attention deficit hyperactivity disorder. In P. J. Accardo, T. A. Blondis, & B. Y. Whitman (Eds.), *Attention deficit disorder and hyperactivity in children* (pp. 85–120). New York: Marcel Dekker.

Bonde, H. V., Andersen, J. P., & Rosenkilde, P. (1994). Nocturnal enuresis: Change of nocturnal voiding pattern during alarm treatment. *Scandinavian Journal of Urology and Nephrology, 28,* 349–352.

Brazelton, T. B. (1962). A child-oriented approach to toilet training. *Pediatrics, 29,* 121–128.

Briere, J. N. (1992). *Child abuse trauma: Theory and treatment of the lasting effects.* Newbury Park, CA: Sage.

Brooks, R. B. (1985). The beginning sessions of child therapy: Of messages and metaphors. *Psychotherapy, 22,* 761–769.

Brooks, R. C., Copen, R. M., Cox, D. J., Morris, J., Borowitz, S., & Sutphen, J. (2000). Review of the treatment literature for encopresis, functional constipation, and stool-toileting refusal. *Annals of Behavioral Medicine, 22,* 260–267.

Campbell, S. B. (1987). Parent-referred problem three-year-olds: Developmental changes in symptoms. *Journal of Child Psychology and Psychiatry, 28,* 835–845.

Campbell, S. B. (1994). Hard-to-manage preschool boys: Externalizing behavior, social competence, and family context at two-year followup. *Journal of Abnormal Child Psychology, 22,* 147–166.

Campbell, S. B. (1995). Behavior problems in preschool children: A review of recent research. *Journal of Child Psychology and Psychiatry, 36,* 113–149.

Campbell, S. B. (1997). Behavior problems in preschool children: Developmental and family issues. In T. H. Ollendick & R. J. Prinz (Eds.), *Advances in clinical child psychology* (Vol. 19, pp. 1–26). New York: Plenum.

Campbell, S. B., & Ewing, L. J. (1990). Follow-up of hard-to-manage preschoolers: Adjustment at age 9 and predictors of continuing symptoms. *Journal of Child Psychology and Psychiatry, 31,* 871–889.

Campbell, S. B., Ewing, L. J., Breaux, A. M., & Szumowski, E. K. (1986). Parent-referred problem three-year-olds: Follow-up at school entry. *Journal of Child Psychology and Psychiatry, 27,* 473–488.

Campbell, S. B., Pierce, E. W., Moore, G., Marakovitz, S., & Newby, K. (1996). Boys' externalizing problems at elementary school age: Pathways from early behavior problems, maternal control, and family stress. *Development and Psychopathology, 8,* 701–719.

Capps, L., Sigman, M., & Mundy, P. (1994). Attachment security in children with autism. *Development and Psychopathology, 6,* 249–261.

Carter, A. S., Garrity-Rokous, F. E., Chazan-Cohen, R., Little, C., & Briggs-Gowan, M. J. (2001). Maternal depression and comorbidity: Predicting early parenting, attachment security, and toddler social–emotional problems and competencies. *Journal of the American Academy of Child and Adolescent Psychiatry, 40,* 18–26.

Chandler, L. A., & Johnson, V. J. (1991). *Using projective techniques with children.* Springfield, IL: Thomas.

Cohen, J. A., Marrarino, A. P., Berliner, L., & Deblinger, E. (2000). Trauma-focused cognitive behavioral therapy for children and adolescents: An empirical update. *Journal of Interpersonal Violence, 15,* 1202–1223.

Collett, B. R., Crowley, S. L., Gimpel, G. A., & Greenson, J. N. (2000). The factor structure of DSM-IV attention deficit–hyperactivity symptoms: A confirmatory factor analysis of the ADHD-SRS. *Journal of Psychoeducational Assessment, 18,* 361–373.

Conduct Problems Prevention Research Group. (1999a). Initial impact of the Fast Track prevention trial for conduct problems: I. The high-risk sample. *Journal of Consulting and Clinical Psychology, 67,* 631–647.

Conduct Problems Prevention Research Group. (1999b). Initial impact of the Fast Track prevention trial for conduct problems: II. Classroom effects. *Journal of Consulting and Clinical Psychology, 67,* 648–657.

Conners, C. K. (1997). *Conners' Rating Scales manual.* North Tonawanda, NY: Multi-Health Systems.

Dadds, M. R., Schwartz, S., Sanders, M. R. (1987). Marital discord and treatment outcome in behavioral treatment of child conduct disorders. *Journal of Consulting and Clinical Psychology, 55,* 396–403.

Deblinger, E., McLeer, S., & Henry, D. (1990). Cognitive behavioral treatment for sexually abused children suffering post-traumatic stress: Preliminary findings. *American Academy of Child and Adolescent Psychiatry, 29,* 747–752.

DuPaul, G. J., & Eckert, T. L. (1994). The effects of social skills curricula: Now you see them, now you don't. *School Psychology Quarterly, 9,* 113–132.

DuPaul, G. J., Power, T. J., Anastopoulos, A. D., & Reid, R. (1998). *ADHD Rating Scale–IV: Checklists, norms, and clinical interpretation.* New York: Guilford Press.

Durand, V. M., Mindell, J., Mapstone, E., & Gernet-Dott, P. (1998). Sleep problems. In T. S. Watson & F. M. Gresham (Eds.), *Handbook of child behavior therapy* (pp. 203–219). New York: Plenum.

Earls, F. (1982). Application of DSM-III in an epidemiological study of preschool children. *American Journal of Psychiatry, 139,* 242–243.

Eddy, J. M., Leve, L. D., & Fagot, B. I. (2001). Coercive family processes: A replication and extension of Patterson's coercion model. *Aggressive Behavior, 27,* 14–25.

Eisenstadt, T. H., Eyberg, S., McNeil, C. B., Newcomb, K., & Funderburk, B. (1993). Parent–child interaction therapy with behavior problem children: Relative effectiveness of two stages and overall treatment outcome. *Journal of Clinical Child Psychology, 22,* 42–51.

Eyberg, S. M., Edwards, D., Boggs, S. R., & Foote, R. (1998). Maintaining the treatment effects of parent training: The role of booster sessions and other maintenance strategies. *Clinical Psychology: Science and Practice, 5,* 544–554.

Eyberg, S. M., & Ross, A. W. (1978). Assessment of child behavior problems: The validation of a new inventory. *Journal of Clinical Child Psychology, 7,* 113–116.

Fletcher, K. E. (2003). Childhood posttraumatic stress disorder. In E. J. Mash & R. A. Barkley (Eds.), *Child psychopathology* (2nd ed., pp. 330–371). New York: Guilford Press.

Forsythe, W. I., & Redmond, A. (1974). Enuresis and spontaneous cure rate: Study of 1,129 enuretics. *Archives of Diseases in Childhood, 49,* 259–269.

France, K. G., Henderson, J. M. T., & Hudson, S. (1996). Fact, act, and tact: A three-stage approach to treating the sleep problems of infants and young children. *Child and Adolescent Psychiatric Clinics of North America, 5,* 581–599.

Friman, P. C., Hoff, K. E., Schnoes, C., Freeman, K. A., Woods, D. W., & Blum, N. (1999). The bedtime pass: An approach to bedtime crying and leaving the room. *Archives of Pediatric and Adolescent Medicine, 153,* 1027–1029.

Garbarino, J., Stott, F., and Faculty of the Erikson Institute. (1992). *What children can tell us.* San Francisco, CA: Jossey-Bass.

Garber, S. W., Garber, M. D., Spizman, R. F. (1992). *Good behavior made easy handbook.* Glastonbury, CT: Great Pond Publishing.

Gil, E. (1991). *The healing power of play: Working with abused children.* New York: Guilford Press.

Glaser, D. (1991). Treatment issues in child sexual abuse. *British Journal of Psychiatry, 159,* 769–782.

Greenspan, S. I., & Greenspan, N. T. (1991). *Clinical interview of the child* (2nd ed.). Washington, DC: American Psychiatric Press.

Gresham, F. M., & Elliot, S. N. (1990). *The Social Skills Rating System.* Circle Pines, MN: American Guidance.

Gresham, F. M., & Lambros, K. M. (1998). Behavioral and functional assessment. In T. S. Watson & F. M. Gresham (Eds.), *Handbook of child behavior therapy* (pp. 3–22). New York: Plenum.

Guevremont, D. C., DuPaul, G. J., & Barkley, R. A. (1993). Behavioral assessment of attention deficit hyperactivity disorder. In J. L. Matson (Ed.), *Handbook of hyperactivity in children* (pp. 150–168). Needham Heights, MA: Allyn & Bacon.

Hammen, C., & Rudolph, K. D. (2003). Childhood mood disorders. In E. J. Mash & R. A. Barkley (Eds.), *Child psychopathology* (2nd ed., pp. 223–278). New York: Guilford Press.

Hanf, C. (1969). *A two-stage program for modifying maternal controlling during mother–child (m-c) interaction.* Paper presented at the annual meeting of the Western Psychological Association, Vancouver, British Columbia.

Hawkins, R. P. (1979). The functions of assessment: Implications for selection and development of devices for assessing repertoires in clinical, educational, and other settings. *Journal of Applied Behavior Analysis, 12,* 501–516.

Heller, T. L., Baker, B. L., Henker, B., & Hinshaw, S. P. (1996). Externalizing behavior and cognitive functioning from preschool to first grade: Stability and predictors. *Journal of Clinical Child Psychology, 25,* 376–387.

Hembree-Kigin, T. L., & McNeil, C. B. (1995). *Parent–child interaction therapy.* New York: Plenum.

Holland, M. L., Gimpel, G. A., & Merrell, K. W. (2001). *ADHD Symptoms Rating Scale (ADHD-SRS).* Wilmington, DE: Wide Range.

Howe, A. C., & Walker, C. E. (1992). Behavioral management of toilet training, enuresis, and encopresis. *Pediatric Clinics of North America, 39,* 413–432.

Huberty, T. J. (1998). Anxiety in children: Information for parents. In A. S. Canter & S. A. Carroll (Eds.), *Helping children at home and school: Handouts from your school psychologist* (pp. 227–229). Bethesda, MD: National Association of School Psychologists.

Huesmann, L. R., Eron, L. D., Lefkowitz, M. M., & Walder, L. O. (1984). Stability of aggression over time and generations. *Developmental Psychology, 20,* 1120–1134.

Hughes, J. N., & Baker, D. B. (1990). *The clinical child interview.* New York: Guilford Press.

Jersild, A. T. (1968). *Child psychology* (6th ed.). Englewood Cliffs, NJ: Prentice-Hall.

Kamphaus, R. W., & Frick, P. J. (1996). *Clinical assessment of child and adolescent personality and behavior.* Boston: Allyn & Bacon.

Kashani, J. H., Horwitz, E., Ray, J. S., & Reid, J. C. (1986). DSM-III diagnostic classification of 100 preschoolers in a child development unit. *Child Psychiatry and Human Development, 16,* 137–147.

Kaslow, N. J., Morris, M. K., & Rehm, L. P. (1998). Childhood depression. In T. R. Kratochwill & R. J. Morris (Eds.), *The practice of child therapy* (3rd ed., pp. 48–90). Boston: Allyn & Bacon.

Kaufman, J., & Henrich, C. (2000). Exposure to violence and early childhood trauma. In C. H. Zeanah (Ed.), *Handbook of infant mental health* (2nd ed., pp. 195–207). New York: Guilford Press.

Kazdin, A. E. (1993). Treatment of conduct disorder: Progress and directions in psychotherapy research. *Development and Psychopathology, 5,* 277–310.

Kazdin, A. E. (1997). Parent management training: Evidence, outcomes, and issues. *Journal of the American Academy of Child and Adolescent Psychiatry, 36,* 1349–1356.

Kazdin, A. E. (2001). *Behavior modification in applied settings* (6th ed.). Belmont, CA: Wadsworth.

Kazdin, A. E., Siegel, T. C., & Bass, D. (1992). Cognitive problem-solving skills training and parent management training in the treatment of antisocial behavior in children. *Journal of Consulting and Clinical Psychology, 60,* 733–747.

Kazdin, A. E., & Wassell, G. (2000). Therapeutic changes in children, parents, and families resulting from treatment of children with conduct disorders. *Journal of the American Academy of Child and Adolescent Psychiatry, 39,* 414–420.

Kedesdy, J. H., & Budd, K. S. (1998). *Childhood feeding disorders: Biobehavioral assessment and intervention.* Baltimore, MD: Brookes.

Keenan, K., Shaw, D., Delliquadri, E., Giovannelli, J., & Walsh, B. (1998). Evidence of the continuity of early problem behaviors: Application of a developmental model. *Journal of Abnormal Child Psychology, 26,* 441–454.

Keenan, K., Shaw, D. S., Walsh, B., Delliquadri, E., & Giovannelli, J. (1997). DSM-III–R disorders in preschool children from low-income families. *Journal of the American Academy of Child and Adolescent Psychiatry, 35,* 620–627.

Keenan, K., & Wakschlag, L. S. (2000). More than the terrible twos: The nature and severity of behavior problems in clinic-referred preschool children. *Journal of Abnormal Child Psychology, 28,* 33–46.

Keenan, K., & Wakschlag, L. S. (2002). Can a valid diagnosis of disruptive behavior disorder be made in preschool children? *American Journal of Psychiatry, 159,* 351–358.

Kehle, T. J., & Bray, M. A. (1998). Selective mutism: A handout for parents and teachers. In A.

S. Canter & S. A. Carroll (Eds.), *Helping children at home and school: Handouts from your school psychologist* (pp. 263–265). Bethesda, MD: National Association of School Psychologists.

Keith, L. K., & Campbell, J. M. (2000). Assessment of social and emotional development in preschool children. In B. A. Bracken (Ed.), *The psychoeducational assessment of preschool children* (3rd ed., pp. 364–382). Boston: Allyn & Bacon.

Kelley, M. L. (1990). *School–home notes: Promoting children's classroom success.* New York: Guilford Press.

Kerr, S., & Jowett, S. (1994). Sleep problems in pre-school children: A review of the literature. *Child: Care, health, and development, 20,* 379–391.

Kerwin, M. E. (1999). Empirically supported treatments in pediatric psychology: Severe feeding problems. *Journal of Pediatric Psychology, 24,* 193–214.

King, N., Tonge, B. J., Mullen, P., Myseron, N., Heyne, D., Rollings, S., & Ollendick, T. H. (2000). Sexually abused children and post-traumatic stress disorder. *Counselling Psychology Quarterly, 13,* 365–375.

Klinger, L. G., Dawson, G., & Renner, P. (2003). Autistic disorder. In E. J. Mash & R. A. Barkley (Eds.), *Child psychopathology* (2nd ed., pp. 409–454). New York: Guilford Press.

Knell, S. M. (2000). Cognitive-behavioral play therapy for childhood fears and phobias. In H. G. Kaduson & C. E. Schaefer (Eds.), *Short-term play therapy for children* (pp. 3–27). New York: Guilford Press.

Koppitz, E. M. (1968). *Psychological evaluation of children's human figure drawings.* New York: Grune & Stratton.

Kuhn, B. R., Marcus, B. A., & Pitner, S. L. (1999). Treatment guidelines for primary non-retentive encopresis and stool toileting refusal. *American Family Physician, 59,* 2171–2178.

Kuhn, B. R., & Weidinger, D. (2000). Interventions for infant and toddler sleep disturbance: A review. *Child and Family Behavior Therapy, 22,* 33–50.

Lahey, B. B., Pelham, W. E., Stein, M. A., Loney, J., Trapani, C., Nugent, K., Kipp, H., Schmidt, E., Lee, S., Cale, M., Gold, E., Hartung, C. M., Willcutt, E., & Baumann, B. (1998). Validity of DSM-IV attention-deficit/hyperactivity disorder for younger children. *Journal of the American Academy of Child and Adolescent Psychiatry, 37,* 695–702.

Lavigne, J. V., Gibbons, R. D., Christoffel, K. K., Arend, R., Rosenbaum, D., Binns, H., Dawson, N., Sobel, H., & Isaacs, C. (1996). Prevalence rates and correlates of psychiatric disorders among preschool children. *Journal of the American Academy of Child and Adolescent Psychiatry, 35,* 204–214.

Linscheid, T. R., Budd, K. S., & Rasnake, L. K. (1995). Pediatric feeding disorders. In M. C. Roberts (Ed.), *Handbook of pediatric psychology* (2nd ed., pp. 501–515). New York: Guilford Press.

Loeber, R., Green, S. M., Lahey, B. B., Frick, P. J., & McBurnett, K. (2000). Findings on disruptive behavior disorders from the first decade of the developmental trends study. *Clinical Child and Family Psychology Review, 3,* 37–60.

Luby, J. L. (2000). Depression. In C. H. Zeanah (Ed), *Handbook of infant mental health* (2nd ed., pp. 382–396). New York: Guilford Press.

Mark, S. D., & Frank, J. D. (1995). Nocturnal enuresis. *British Journal of Urology, 75,* 427–434.

Mathiesen, K. S., & Sanson, A. (2000). Dimensions of early childhood behavior problems: Stability and predictors of change from 18 to 30 months. *Journal of Abnormal Child Psychology, 28,* 15–31.

Mayhall, P. D., & Norgard, K. E. (1983). *Child abuse and neglect: Sharing responsibility.* New York: Macmillan.

McCarney, S. B. (1995a). *The Attention Deficit Disorders Evaluation Scale, home version, technical manual.* Columbia, MO: Hawthorne.

McCarney, S. B. (1995b). *The Attention Deficit Disorders Evaluation Scale, school version, technical manual.* Columbia, MO: Hawthorne.

McCarney, S. B. (1995c). *The Early Childhood Attention Deficit Disorders Evaluation Scale, home version, technical manual.* Columbia, MO: Hawthorne.

McCarney, S. B. (1995d). *The Early Childhood Attention Deficit Disorders Evaluation Scale, school version, technical manual.* Columbia, MO: Hawthorne.

McGee, R., Partridge, F., Williams, S., & Silva, P. A. (1991). A twelve-year follow-up of preschool hyperactive children. *Journal of the American Academy of Child and Adolescent Psychiatry, 30,* 224–232.

McGinnis, E., & Goldstein, A. P. (1990). *Skillstreaming in early childhood: Teaching prosocial skills to the preschool and kindergarten child.* Champaign, IL: Research Press.

McGoey, K. E., & DuPaul, G. J. (2000). Token reinforcement and response cost procedures: Reducing the disruptive behavior of preschool children with Attention-Deficit/Hyperactivity Disorder. *School Psychology Quarterly, 15,* 330–343.

McMahon, R. J., & Estes, A. M. (1997). Conduct problems. In E. J. Mash & L. G. Terdal (Eds.), *Assessment of childhood disorders* (3rd ed., pp. 130–193). New York: Guilford Press.

Merrell, K. M. (1994). *Preschool and Kindergarten Behavior Scales.* Austin, TX: Pro-Ed.

Merrell, K. W. (1999). *Behavioral, social, and emotional assessment of children and adolescents.* Mahwah, NJ: Erlbaum.

Mindell, J. A. (1993). Sleep disorders in children. *Health Psychology, 12,* 151–162.

Mindell, J. A. (1996). Treatment of child and adolescent sleep disorders. *Child and Adolescent Psychiatric Clinics of North America, 5,* 741–751.

Mindell, J. A. (1999). Empirically supported treatments in pediatric psychology: Bedtime refusal and night wakings in young children. *Journal of Pediatric Psychology, 24,* 465–481.

Morris, R. J., & Kratochwill, T. R. (1998). Childhood fears and phobias. In R. J. Morris & T. R. Kratochwill (Eds.), *The practice of child therapy* (3rd ed., pp. 91–131). Boston: Allyn & Bacon.

Motta, R. W., & Basile, D. M. (1998). Pica. In L. Phelps (Ed.), *Health-related disorders in children and adolescents: A guidebook for understanding and educating* (pp. 524–527). Washington, DC: American Psychological Association.

National Research Council. (2001). *Educating children with autism.* Washington, DC: National Academy Press.

O'Brien, S., Repp, A. C., Williams, G. E., & Christophersen, E. R. (1991). Pediatric feeding disorders. *Behavior Modification, 15,* 394–418.

Olafson, E., & Boat, B. W. (2000). Long-term management of the sexually abused child: Considerations and challenges. In R. M. Reece (Ed.), *Treatment of child abuse: Common ground for mental health, medical, and legal practitioners* (pp. 14–35). Baltimore, MD: Johns Hopkins University Press.

Ollendick, T. H., & King, N. J. (1998). Empirically supported treatments for children with phobic and anxiety disorders: Current status. *Journal of Clinical Child Psychology, 27,* 156–167.

Paige, L. Z. (1998). School phobia/school avoidance/school refusal: A handout for parents and teachers. In A. S. Canter & S. A. Carroll (Eds.), *Helping children at home and school: Handouts from your school psychologist* (pp. 259–262). Bethesda, MD: National Association of School Psychologists.

Patterson, G. R. (1982). *Coercive family process.* Eugene, OR: Castalia.

Pfiffner, L. J., & Barkley, R. A. (1998). Treatment of ADHD in school settings. In R. A. Barkley, *Attention deficit hyperactivity disorder: A handbook for diagnosis and treatment* (2nd ed., pp. 458–490). New York: Guilford Press.

Phillips, P. L., Greenson, J. N., Collett, B. R., & Gimpel, G. A. (2002). Assessing ADHD symptoms in preschool children: Use of the ADHD Symptoms Rating Scale. *Early Education and Development,13,* 283–299.

Piaget, J. (1983). Piaget's theory. In P. H. Mussen (Series Ed.) & W. Kessen (Vol. Ed.) *Handbook of child psychology: Vol. 1. History, theory, and methods* (4th ed., pp. 103–128). New York: Wiley.

Pierce, E. W., Ewing, L. J., & Campbell, S. B. (1999). Diagnostic status and symptomatic behavior of hard-to-manage preschool children in middle childhood and early adolescence. *Journal of Clinical Child Psychology, 28,* 44–57.

Pisterman, S., McGrath, P., Firestone, P., Goodman, J. T., Webster, I., & Mallory, R. (1989). Outcome of parent-mediated treatment with preschoolers with attention deficit disorder with hyperactivity. *Journal of Consulting and Clinical Psychology, 57,* 628–635.

Reynolds, C. R., & Kamphaus, R. W. (1992). *Behavior assessment system for children.* Circle Pines, MN: American Guidance.

Reynolds, L. K., & Kelley, M. L. (1997). The efficacy of a response cost-based treatment package for managing aggressive behavior in preschoolers. *Behavior Modification, 21,* 216–230.

Ross, D. M., & Ross, S. A. (1982). *Hyperactivity: Current issues, research, and theory* (2nd ed.). New York: Wiley.

Saklofske, D. H., Janzen, H. L., Hildebrand, D. K., & Kaufmann, L. (1998). Depression in children: A handout for parents and teachers. In A. S. Canter & S. A. Carroll (Eds.), *Helping children at home and school: Handouts from your school psychologist.* Bethesda, MD: National Association of School Psychologists.

Sattler, J. M. (1998). *Clinical and forensic interviewing of children and families.* San Diego: Author.

Saywitz, K. J., Mannarino, A. P., Berliner, L., & Cohen, J. A. (2000). Treatment for sexually abused children and adolescents. *American Psychologist, 55,* 1040–1049.

Scheeringa, M. S.,& Gaensbauer T. J. (2000). Posttraumatic stress disorder. In C. H. Zeanah (Ed.), *Handbook of infant mental health* (2nd ed., pp. 369–381). New York: Guilford Press.

Schroeder, C. S., & Gordon, B. N. (2002). *Assessment and treatment of childhood problems: A clinician's guide* (2nd ed.). New York: Guilford Press.

Schuhmann, E. M., Foote, R. C., Eyberg, S. M., Boggs, S. R., & Algina, J. (1998). Efficacy of parent–child interaction therapy: Interim report of a randomized trial with short-term maintenance. *Journal of Clinical Child Psychology, 27*, 34–45.

Schulman, S. L., Colish, Y., von Zuben, F. C., & Kodman-Jones, C. (2000). Effectiveness of treatments for nocturnal enuresis in a heterogeneous population. *Clinical Pediatrics, 39*, 359–364.

Schwartz, C. E., Snidman, N., & Kagan, J. (1999). Adolescent social anxiety as an outcome of inhibited temperament in childhood. *Journal of the American Academy of Child and Adolescent Psychiatry, 38*, 1008–1015.

Serketich, W. J., & Dumas, J. E. (1996). The effectiveness of behavioral parent training to modify antisocial behavior in children: A meta-analysis. *Behavior Therapy, 27*, 171–186.

Shaw, D. S., Keenan, K., Vondra, J. I., Delliquadri, E., & Giovannelli, J. (1997). Antecedents of preschool children(s internalizing problems: A longitudinal study of low-income families. *Journal of the American Academy of Child and Adolescent Psychiatry, 36*, 1760–1767.

Shaw, D. S., Owens, E. B., Giovannelli, J., & Winslow, E. B. (2001). Infant and toddler pathways leading to early externalizing disorders. *Journal of the American Academy of Child and Adolescent Psychiatry, 40*, 36–43.

Shaw, D. S., Owens, E. B., Vondra, J. I., Keenan, K., & Winslow, E. B. (1996). Early risk factors and pathways of early disruptive behavior problems. *Development and Psychopathology, 8*, 679–699.

Shelby, J. (2000). Brief therapy with traumatized children: A developmental perspective. In H. G. Kaudsoon & C. E. Schaefer (Eds.), *Short-term play therapy for children* (pp. 69–104). New York: Guilford Press.

Shelton, T. L., Barkley, R. A., Crosswait, C., Moorehouse, M., Fletcher, K., Barrett, S., Jenkins, L., & Metevia, L. (2000). Multimethod psychoeducational intervention for preschool children with disruptive behavior: Two-year post-treatment follow-up. *Journal of Abnormal Child Psychology, 28*, 253–266.

Shonkoff, J. P., & Meisels, S. J. (1990). Early childhood intervention: The evolution of a concept. In S. J. Meisels & J. P. Shonkoff (Eds.), *Handbook of early childhood intervention.* New York: Cambridge University Press.

Sonuga-Barke, E. J. S., Daley, D., Thompson, M., Laver-Bradbury, C., & Weeks, A. (2001). Parent-based therapies for preschool attention deficit/hyperactivity disorder: A randomized, controlled trial with a community sample. *Journal of the American Academy of Child and Adolescent Psychiatry, 40*, 402–408.

Stallard, P. (1993). The behavior of 3-year-old children: Prevalence and parental perception of problem behaviour: A research note. *Journal of Child Psychology and Psychiatry and Allied Disciplines, 34*, 413–421.

State of California Department of Social Services. (1997). *The California child abuse and neglect reporting law.* Pamphlet distributed by the State of California Department of Social Services: Office of Child Abuse Prevention, Sacramento, CA.

Stores, G. (2001). *A clinical guide to sleep disorders in children and adolescents.* Cambridge, UK: Cambridge University Press.

Sue, D. W., & Sue, S. (1990). *Counseling the culturally different* (2nd ed.). New York: Wiley.

Sullivan, M. A., & O'Leary, S. G. (1990). Maintenance following reward and response cost token programs. *Behavior Therapy, 21*, 139–151.

Tanguay, P. E. (2000). Pervasive development disorders: A 10-year review. *Journal of the American Academy of Child and Adolescent Psychiatry, 39,* 1079–1095.

Thiedke, C. C. (2001). Sleep disorders and sleep problems in children. *American Family Physician, 63,* 277–284.

Thomas, J. M., & Guskin, K. A. (2001). Disruptive behavior in young children: What does it mean? *Journal of the American Academy of Child and Adolescent Psychiatry, 40,* 44–51.

Tremblay, R. E., Pagani-Kurtz, L., Masse, L. C., Vitaro, F., & Pihl, R. O. (1995). A bimodal preventive intervention for disruptive kindergarten boys: Its impact through mid-adolescence. *Journal of Consulting and Clinical Psychology, 63,* 560–568.

Turner, H. S., & Watson, T. S. (1999). Consultants guide for the use of time-out in the preschool and elementary classroom. *Psychology in the Schools, 36,* 135–148

U.S. Department of Health and Human Services, National Center on Child Abuse and Neglect. (1997). *Child maltreatment 1995: Reports for the states to the national center on child abuse and neglect data system.* Washington, DC: U.S. Government Printing Office.

Wakschlag, L. S., & Keenan, K. (2001). Clinical significance and correlates of disruptive behavior in environmentally at-risk preschoolers. *Journal of Child Clinical Psychology, 30,* 262–275.

Walker, C. E. (1995). Elimination disorders: Enuresis and encopresis. In M .C. Roberts (Ed.), *Handbook of pediatric psychology* (2nd ed., pp. 537–557). New York: Guilford Press.

Walker, H. M., Severson, H. H., & Feil, E. G. (1995). *The Early Screening Project: A proven child find process.* Longmont, CO: Sopris West.

Warren, S. L., Huston, L., Egeland, B., & Sroufe, A. L. (1997). Child and adolescent anxiety disorders and early attachment. *Journal of the American Academy of Child and Adolescent Psychiatry, 36,* 637–644.

Webster-Stratton, C. (1984). Randomized trial of two parent-training programs for families with conduct-disordered children. *Journal of Consulting and Clinical Psychology, 52,* 666–678.

Webster-Stratton, C. (1994). Advancing videotape parent training: A comparison study. *Journal of Consulting and Clinical Psychology, 62,* 583–593.

Webster-Stratton, C. (1996). Early-onset conduct problems: Does gender make a difference? *Journal of Consulting and Clinical Psychology, 64,* 540–551.

Webster-Stratton, C. (1998). Preventing conduct problems in Head Start children: Strengthening parenting competencies. *Journal of Consulting and Clinical Psychology, 66,* 715–730.

Webster-Stratton, C., & Hammond, M. (1997). Treating children with early-onset conduct problems: A comparison of child and parent training interventions. *Journal of Consulting and Clinical Psychology, 65,* 93–109.

Webster-Stratton, C., & Hancock, L. (1998). Training for parents of young children with conduct problems: Content, methods, and therapeutic procedures. In J. M. Briesmeister & C. E. Schaefer (Eds.), *Handbook of parent training: Parents as co-therapists for children's behavior problems* (2nd ed., pp. 98–152). New York: Wiley.

Webster-Stratton, C., Reid, M. J., & Hammond, M. (2001). Preventing conduct problems, promoting social competence: A parent and teacher training partnership in Head Start. *Journal of Clinical Child Psychology, 30,* 283–302.

Index

Abuse and neglect, 7–8. See also
    Child abuse; Neglect
Acting-out problems. See
    Externalizing problems
Acute stress disorder, 7
ADHD. See Attention-deficit/
    hyperactivity disorder
ADHD Rating Scale-IV, 40–41
ADHD-Symptoms Rating Scale, 40
Alarms, for enuresis treatment, 117,
    122, 123f, 124f, 125
Antecedents, defined, 42, 55f
Anxiety
    versus fear, 87
    separation, 88–89. See also
        Separation anxiety disorder
Anxiety disorders, 4–5
    parent handout for, 98f
    prevalence of, 12
    symptoms of, 87
Arousal disorders, 143–146
Asperger's disorder, 9
Assessment, 19–49
    direct observation in, 41–49
        formal, 49
        structured, 42–48
    forms for, 21f, 23f–26f
    functional, 46
    interviews in
        with parents/caregivers, 20–28
        with teachers/daycare workers,
            28–29
        with young children, 29–35
    rating scales in, 35–41
        ADHD-Rating Scale-IV, 40–
            41
        ADHD-Symptoms Rating
            Scale, 40
        Attention Deficit Disorder
            Evaluation Scale, 39–40

Behavior Assessment System for
    Children, 36–37, 37t
Child Behavior Checklist, 35–
    36, 36t
Conners' Rating Scales, 37–38,
    38t
Eyberg Child Behavior
    Inventory, 38–39
Preschool and Kindergarten
    Behavior Scales, 38
Social Skills Rating System, 39
Teacher's Report Form, 35–36,
    36t
recent developments in, 19–20
Attention
    positive, 58f–59f
    selective, 76
Attention Deficit Disorder Evaluation
    Scale, 39–40
Attention-deficit/hyperactivity
    disorder, 2–3, 2t
    defined, 3
    prevalence of, 11–12
    response-cost programs and, 76–77
    treatment of. See Externalizing
        problems, treatment of
Autism, 8–9

B

Bedwetting. See Enuresis
Behavior
    ABCs of, 55
    appropriate, providing privileges
        for, 69f–70f
    inappropriate, losing privileges for,
        69f–70f
    observable, defining, 42
Behavior Assessment System for
    Children, 36–37, 36t

Behavior log
    for functional analysis, 48f
    for home behavior, 47f
Behavior problems
    assessment of. See Assessment
    differing perceptions of, 20, 22
    managing, in public places, 73f
    predictors of, 14–18, 14t
        externalizing, 14–16, 14t
        internalizing, 14t, 15t, 17–18
    stability of, 13–14
Behavior rating scales, 19
Behavioral principles, 54, 55f–56f
Behavioral, social, and emotional
    problems. See Disorders;
        specific disorders
Behavioral interventions. See
    Interventions
Breathing
    deep, for phobia treatment, 92, 94
    slow, 94

C

Caregivers, interviewing, 20, 22, 22t,
    27–28
CD. See Conduct disorders
Central tendency, error of, 41
Child abuse, 147–160. See also
        Posttraumatic stress disorder
    effects of, 148–149, 152
        physical, 149
        psychological, 149, 152
    interventions for victims of, 152–
        155
    legal requirements for reporting,
        148
    neglect, 148
    physical, 147
    psychological, 148–149

Child abuse *(cont.)*
 resources for, 159–160
 risk factors for, 158–159
 sexual, 147–148
 signs and symptoms of, 150f–151f
Child Behavior Checklist, 35–36, 36t
Child development, obtaining
  information on, 27
Child intake form, 23f–26f
Child protective agencies, reporting
  to, 148
Childhood disintegrative disorder, 9
Children
 backgrounds of, 22
 information provided by, 19–20
 interviews with, 29–35
  context of, 32–34
  developmental issues and, 29–
   30
  information gathering in, 30–32
  mental status exam in, 34–35
  rapport building in, 30–32, 32t
  theories about, 29
Child's Game, 54
Classroom, posting rules in, 75–76
Cognitive functioning, obtaining
  information on, 27
Cognitive-behavioral therapy
 for child abuse victims, 155
 for PTSD, 156–158
Commands
 effective, 60, 62–63, 63f
 rationales for, 60, 62
Conditioning, operant, principles of,
  54–56
Conduct disorders, 2, 2t, 4
 defined, 4
 treatment of. See Externalizing
  problems, treatment of
Conners' Rating Scales, 37–38, 38t
Consent form, 21f
Consequences, defined, 42, 55
Constipation, in retentive encopresis,
  125–126
Contingency contracting, 67, 69f–70f,
  71f, 72
Contingency management, for phobia
  treatment, 98f, 100
Contracting, 105
 contingency, 67, 69f–70f, 71f, 72
Coping skills, training in, 157
Cultural issues
 in child discipline, 148
 in child interviews, 33–34

D

Daycare workers, role with depressed
  children, 112
Deep breathing, for phobia
  treatment, 92, 94

Depression, 6, 107–112
 preventing, 108
 treating, 108–112
Desensitization, systematic
 for phobia treatment, 98f
 for specific phobias, 91–98
Development. See Child
  development; Emotional
  development
Developmental disorders, pervasive,
  8–10
Diagnostic and Statistical Manual of
  Mental Disorders, 4th ed.
 multiaxial approach of, 11
Differential reinforcement, 56
Direct observation, 41–49
 coding procedures for, 43t
 informal, by parents/teachers, 45–
  46
 naturalistic, 42
 setting variables in, 42–43
 structured, 42–48
 informal, 43–44
Discipline
 appropriate, 60, 62–63
 cultural issues in, 148
Disorders
 abuse and neglect, 7–8
 developmental, 8–10
 externalizing, 2–4, 2t. See also
  Externalizing problems
 feeding, 7
 internalizing, 2t, 4–6. See also
  Internalizing problems
 introduction to, 2–18
 prevalence/definition issues and,
  10–12
 selective mutism, 6
 sleep, 7
 toileting, 6–7
Dolls, anatomically correct, 31
Drawing techniques, building rapport
  with, 31
Duration recording, 44
Dysthymic disorder, 6

E

Early Childhood Attention Deficit
  Disorders Evaluation Scale,
  40
Early interventions, increased
  emphasis on, 19
Early Screening Project, 49
Echolalia, 8
Emotional abuse, signs and symptoms
  of, 151f
Emotional development, obtaining
  information on, 28
Emotive imagery, for phobia
  treatment, 96–97

Encopresis, 6–7, 125–130
 diagnosis of, 125
 nonretentive, 127, 130
 retentive, 125–127
 treatment, 125–127, 130
 treatment guidelines for, 128f
 treatment log for, 129f
Enuresis, 6–7, 116–125
 diagnosis of, 116
 diurnal, 116
 nocturnal, 116, 122
 prevalence of, 116
 treatment of, 116, 122
 with alarms, 117, 122, 123f,
  124f, 125
 daytime logs in, 118f, 119f
 nighttime logs in, 120f, 121f
Error variance, in rating scales, 41
Escape, 55–56
Event/frequency recording, 43–44
Everyday problems, 114–146
 feeding/eating-related, 130–135
 sleep-related, 135–146
 toileting-related, 114–130
Externalizing problems, 2–4, 2t. See
  also Attention-deficit/
  hyperactivity disorder;
  Conduct disorders;
  Oppositional defiant
  disorder
 treatment of, 50–85
 parent training in, 51–75
 prevention/intervention
  programs in, 82–84
 school-based programs in, 75–
  80
 social skills interventions in,
  80–82
Extinction burst, defined, 56f
Eyberg Child Behavior Inventory,
  38–39
Eye contact, cultural perspectives on,
  34

F

Families. See also Parent training;
  Parenting; Parents
 at-risk, for child abuse, 158–160
 treatment of, in abuse situations,
  153
Family relationships, information on,
  22
Fast Track program, 83
Fear
 versus anxiety, 87
 characteristics of, 86–87
 symptoms of, 87
Fear hierarchy, 91–92, 93f, 94t
Fecal impaction, encopresis and, 125–
  126

Feeding/eating disorders, 7, 130–135
    interview questions for assessing,
        131, 131t
    mealtime problems, guidelines for
        parents, 133f
    organic component in, 131
Feelings charts, 110f, 111f
Food, reinforcement with, 133f

G

GAD. See Generalized anxiety
    disorders
Games, for reinforcing appropriate
    behaviors, 54, 57
Generalized anxiety disorders,
    defined, 5
Genetic mutations, in Rett's disorder, 10
Gradual exposure, for PTSD, 157

H

Halo effect, 41
Home-school notes, 78, 79f, 80

I

Imagery, for phobia treatment, 96
Information, confidential, consent
    form for obtaining, 21f
Instrument variance, 41
Intake form, 23f–26f
Interests, obtaining information
    about, 28
Internalizing problems, 2t, 4–6. See
    also Anxiety disorders;
    Depression
    overview of, 86–89
    prevalence of, 11–12
    symptoms of, 86
    treatment of, 86–113
        anxiety problems, 89–107
        depressive symptoms, 107–112
Interval recording, 44, 45f
Interventions
    for child abuse, 152–155
    early, programs for, 82–84
    social skills, 80–82
Interviews, 20–35
    leading versus nonleading
        questions in, 33
    with parents/caregivers, 20, 22,
        22t, 27–28
    with teachers/daycare workers, 28–
        29
    with young children, 29–35
        context of, 32–34
        developing rapport in, 30–32,
            32t
        mental status examination in,
            34–35

K

Kindergarten
    behavioral interventions in, 75–80
    prevention/early intervention
        programs for, 83

L

Leniency/severity, error of, 41

M

Medical history, 27
Mental health issues, assessment of.
    See Assessment
Mental status examination, 34–35
Modeling, for phobia treatment, 98f, 99
Momentary time sampling, 44
Motivation, parental, 52–53
Muscle relaxation. See Relaxation
    techniques
Mutism, selective. See Selective mutism

N

Negative reinforcement,
        characteristics of, 55f–56f
Neglect, 148
    risk factors for, 158–159
    signs and symptoms of, 150f–151f
    symptoms of, 149
Night terrors, 144, 145f, 146
    definition and intervention, 145f
Nightmares
    definition and intervention, 145f
    versus sleep terrors, 144

O

Observation. See Direct observation
Obsessive-compulsive disorder, 5
OCD. See Obsessive-compulsive
    disorder
ODD. See Oppositional defiant
    disorder
Operant conditioning, principles of, 54–56
Oppositional defiant disorder, 2–4, 2t
    defined, 3
    prevalence of, 11–12
    treatment of. See Externalizing
        problems, treatment of

P

Panic disorder, 6
Parent training
    for management of externalizing
        problems, 51–75
        appropriate use of, 52–53
        behavioral principles in, 54–56

effective command/appropriate
    discipline phase of, 60–72
factors affecting, 52–53
generalization/skill maintenance
    phase of, 72–74
group setting for, 74–75
overview of, 51–52
positive reinforcement phase of,
    54, 57–60
video tape-based, 84
Parenting, cultural issues in, 148
Parents
    of child experiencing PTSD, 156–
        157
    of child with eating disorders, 131–
        132, 131t, 133f
    of child with sleep terrors, 144,
        145f, 146
    communication with, through
        home-school notes, 78, 79f, 80
    concerns of, 10
    of depressed child, 108–109, 112
    enuresis training guidelines for,
        122, 123f, 125
    informal observations by, 45–46
    interviewing, 20, 22, 22t, 27–28
    motivation of, 52–53
    in phobia treatment, 97
    preventing child abuse by, 158–160
Peer relationships, obtaining
    information on, 27
Pervasive developmental disorders,
    8–10
Phobias, 5–6
    specific. See Specific phobias
Physical abuse, interviewing child
    about, 31
Pica, 7
    characteristics and treatment of,
        134
Play activities, for building rapport,
    31–32, 32t
Playtime homework sheet, 61f
Positive reinforcement, 54–60
    for appropriate eating behaviors,
        132
    characteristics of, 55f
    for depressed children, 109, 112
Posttraumatic stress disorder, 7–8, 89,
    152, 156–158
    prevention of, 158–160
    treatment of, 156–158
Praise, 76
    examples of, 59f
Preschool, behavioral interventions
    in, 75–80
Preschool and Kindergarten Behavior
    Scales, 38
Prevention
    of child abuse, 158–160
    programs for, 82–84

Privileges
    behavior management with, 67,
        69f–70f, 71f, 72
    worksheet for, 71f
Problems. See Everyday problems;
        Externalizing problems;
        Internalizing problems
Problem-solving skills, for social
        situations, 80–82
Progressive muscle relaxation, for
        phobia treatment, 94, 95f, 96
Psychiatric history, 27
Psychoeducation, 157
Psychological abuse, 148
    signs of, 149, 152
PTSD. See Posttraumatic stress
        disorder
Public places, managing behavior
        problems in, 73f
Punishment, types of, 56f

R

Rapport, building, 20, 28–29, 30–32,
        32t
Rating scales, 35–41
    limitations of, 41
Reactive attachment disorder, 8, 152
Recording procedures
    duration, 44
    event/frequency, 43–44
    form for, 45f
    interval, 44, 45f
    momentary time sampling, 44
Reflections, examples of, 58f
Reinforcement
    differential, 56
    negative, 55f–56f
    positive. See Positive
        reinforcement
Relaxation techniques
    for anxiety problems, 105
    for phobia treatment, 94, 95f, 96
    for PTSD, 156–158
Release-of-information form, 20, 21f,
        29
Response bias, in rating scales, 41
Response-cost programs, 76–77
Retention-control training, 122
Rett's disorder, 9–10
Reward programs, 72, 74
Rewards, for appropriate eating
        behaviors, 133f
Rules, posting, 75–76

Rumination, 7
    characteristics and treatment of,
        134–135

S

SAD. See Separation anxiety disorder
Safety
    of child abuse victims, 152–153
    psychological, 153–154
School functioning, obtaining
        information on, 27
School refusal. See Separation anxiety
Selective attention, 76
Selective mutism, 6, 105–107
    causes and prevention of, 105–106
    diagnosis of, 105
    treatment of, 106–107
Self-talk, positive, 105
    for phobia treatment, 98f, 99
Separation anxiety disorder, 4–5, 88–
        89, 100–105
    defined, 4
    parent handout on, 103f
    preventing, 101
    treating, 101–102, 104–105
Sexual abuse, 148
    interviewing child about, 31
    providing child with information
        about, 157
    signs and symptoms of, 150f
    symptoms of, 149
Skills, social, interventions for, 80–82
Skillstreaming program, 80–81, 84
Sleep problems, 7, 135–146
    arousal-related, 143–146
    assessment of, 135
    consequences of, 135
    extinction-based interventions for,
        141–143
    in initiating sleep, 136, 141
    interview questions for parents, 136t
    solutions to, 139f–140f
Sleep terrors, 144, 145f, 146
    defined, 145f
Sleepwalking, definition and
        intervention, 145f, 146
Social skills, interventions for, 80–82
Social Skills Rating System, 39
Speaking behaviors, shaping/
        generalization of, 106
Specific phobias, 88
    preventing, 90
    treating, 90–100

Speech disorders, in autism, 8
Spiders, phobia about, 91–98
Statements
    child-directed, examples of, 58f
    directive, avoiding, 59f
Sticker charts, 105
Story-telling, 31
Stress disorders, 7–8
Systematic desensitization, for phobia
        treatment, 98f

T

Talents, obtaining information about,
        28
Target behavior, 42
Teachers
    informal observations by, 45–46
    role with depressed children, 112
Teacher's Report Form, 35–36, 36t
Temporal variance, 41
Therapist, role of, in therapy for child
        abuse victim, 153–154
Time-In, 54
Time-out
    guidelines for, 62, 64f–65f, 77–78
    questions frequently asked about,
        65
Time-out homework sheet, 68f
Toilet training
    child-oriented method of, 115–
        116
    one-day method of, 115
    problems with, 114–116
Toileting, problems with, 6–7, 114–
        130
    encopresis, 125–130
    enuresis, 116–125
    in training, 114–116
Toileting refusal, 127, 130
Token economy systems, 67, 76–77
Toys
    for child abuse victims, 154
    for reinforcing appropriate
        behaviors, 54, 57
Training trips, 72
Trauma. See also Posttraumatic stress
        disorder
    obtaining information about, 28
    types of, 156–157

W

Webster-Stratton, Carolyn, 74–75